Smart Guide™

to

Healing Back Pain

About Smart Guides™

Welcome to Smart Guides. Each Smart Guide is created as a written conversation with a learned friend; a skilled and knowledgeable author guides you through the basics of the subject, selecting the most important points and skipping over anything that's not essential. Along the way, you'll also find smart inside tips and strategies that distinguish this from other books on the topic.

Within each chapter you'll find a number of recurring features to help you find your way through the information and put it to work for you. Here are the user-friendly elements you'll encounter and what they mean:

The Keys

Each chapter opens by highlighting in overview style the most important concepts in the pages that follow.

Smart Move

Here's where you will learn opinions and recommendations from experts and professionals in the field.

Street Smarts

This feature presents smart ways in which people have dealt with related issues and shares their secrets for success.

Smart Sources

Each of these sidebars points the way to more and authoritative information on the topic, from organizations, corporations, publications, web sites, and more.

Smart Definition

Terminology and key concepts essential to your mastering the subject matter are clearly explained in this feature.

F.Y.I.

Related facts, statistics, and quick points of interest are noted here.

What Matters, What Doesn't

Part of learning something new involves distinguishing the most relevant information from conventional wisdom or myth. This feature helps focus your attention on what really matters.

The Bottom Line

The conclusion to each chapter, here is where the lessons learned in each section are summarized so you can revisit the most essential information of the text.

One of the main objectives of the *Smart Guide to Healing Back Pain* is not only to better inform you about the available treatments for back pain, but to educate you about the causes of the pain as well as the preventive measures that can be taken to avoid the discomfort of reinjury.

Smart Guide™
to
Healing Back Pain

Carole Bodger

CADER BOOKS

John Wiley & Sons, Inc.

New York • Chichester • Weinheim • Brisbane • Singapore • Toronto

The information contained in this book is not intended to serve as a replacement for professional medical advice. Any use of the information in this book is at the reader's discretion. The author and the publisher specifically disclaim any and all liability arising directly or indirectly from the use or application of any information contained in this book. A health-care professional should be consulted regarding your specific situation.

Images on pages 10, 11, 13, and 15 are from MediClip, *Human Anatomy 1, 2, 3;* 1996; Lippincott Williams & Wilkins; used with permission. The "Revised Physical Activity Readiness Questionnaire," on page 109, reprinted from the 1994 revised version of *Physical Activity Readiness Questionnaire (PAR-Q and YOU);* the PAR-Q and YOU is a copyrighted pre-exercise screen owned by the Canadian Society for Exercise Physiology. "The McKenzie Exercises," on pages 118–119, from *Treat Your Own Back,* by Robin McKenzie; used with permission of the McKenzie Institute and Spinal Publications New Zealand Ltd.

Library of Congress Cataloging-in-Publication Data:
Bodger, Carole.
Smart guide to healing back pain / Carole Bodger.
p.   cm.
ISBN 0-471-35649-2 (pbk.)
1. Backache. I. Title.
RD771.B217B63   1999
617.5'64—DC21   99-29977

Printed in the United States of America

10 9 8 7 6 5 4 3 2 1

Contents

Introduction

Back pain is a life-changer. It changes the way we move, the things we do, and the manner in which we do them. But it doesn't have to be a life-stopper by any means. Whether you suffer from a dull ache that seems to have had no beginning and is never going to end or periodically grapple with ferocious attacks of sudden anguish, you can take steps to relieve the torment and lessen its negative impact on your life. We hope this book will help.

We start with a look at who's most susceptible to becoming a back-pain sufferer and what can put a person at risk, and move on to a simplified anatomy lesson about the incredibly complex network of bone and tissue summed up in the four-letter word "back." In chapters 2 and 3 we let you in on when you have the greatest likelihood of running into trouble and how to better your odds, as well as when you should see a doctor. The most commonly used tests for diagnosing the cause of pain, and some of the problems that might be detected are discussed next. Chapter 4 explores how the ways in which you move—or stay still—can play a significant role in back health, and suggests an array of preventive, back-strengthening exercises as well as exercises to help relieve pain that has already begun.

In the second half of this book we move on to treatment methods and options, from over-the-counter pills and unguents to high-tech surgical procedures. Chapter 5 reviews the many modes of relief that are available, including prescription and nonprescription drugs, electrical stimulation therapies, and pain-numbing injections. Chapter 6 provides an overview of the numerous surgical approaches to which you might turn when other methods fall short, and is followed by a chapter on popular alternative approaches to healing—such as chiropractic, acupuncture, and mind-body techniques—being used by millions today.

We conclude with a window-shopper's guide to the many products now on the market to help prevent and ease back pain, from body-contoured pillows to gadgets and gizmos that suspend you upside down, with a few words of caution on how to be a good consumer.

We wish we could promise you a "cure" to back pain, but if we did we wouldn't be telling the truth. In many cases, back pain will occur no matter how careful you are to prevent it, and it does have a likelihood of recurring once it's first appeared. The good news is that the great majority of it is preventable. By learning how to strengthen your back bones and muscles and increase your flexibility, by becoming aware of how to move and how not to and knowing what to do to help yourself when back pain does strike, you can lessen the frequency and severity of the pain.

CHAPTER 1

....

Back Basics

THE KEYS

• Back pain is among the most common physical maladies of modern life.

• Lifestyle and other factors affect our susceptibility to back injury and pain.

• A complex network of bones, muscles, ligaments, and nerves, the spinal system functions in more ways than we might expect.

• Back trouble isn't always where we think we'd find it.

Back pain can interfere with every movement, every moment of our waking and less-often-sleeping lives, restricting our activities and monopolizing our attention.

It doesn't have to. In many cases the pain can be eradicated; in others the volume can be turned down. In the best case scenario, back pain can be prevented using simple, precautionary measures within everyone's reach.

Everybody's Enemy

In North America, more people see doctors for back pain than for any other medical ailment, with the exception of colds and upper respiratory complaints, and it's a leading cause of hospitalization and surgery. Low back pain is one of the most frequent problems treated by orthopedic surgeons, according to the American Academy of Orthopaedic Surgeons (AAOS), based in Rosemont, Illinois; and, according to "Women: Work and Health," a Department of Health and Human Services report on the health and well-being of America's working women, for both women *and* men, job-related injuries most frequently affect the back.

An equal opportunity affliction, back pain does not confine itself to men doing hard physical labor in blue-collar jobs. Nurses rank second only to heavy-industry workers in the number of people suffering back pain, reports AAOS. Mothers of newborns, men and women taking care of elderly parents, and other caregivers are common victims.

The good news: as many as one-third of patients with back pain are symptom free within a week, and 90 percent of the time the problem resolves in less than two months. More good news: most cases are acute; only 1 percent of back pain sufferers become chronically disabled. The best news: through relatively modest changes in lifestyle, sufferers can recover faster and better and reduce the likelihood of harming their backs again, and everyone can learn to avoid hurting their backs in the first place.

Do You Fit the Profile of the Back Pain Sufferer?

As the statistics amply demonstrate, back pain can strike any of us: male or female, young or old. The problem can stem from physical injury, disease, emotional duress, poor posture, an inherited congenital flaw, an unhealthy lifestyle, or any combination thereof. With all these possible causes and perhaps others that research has not yet discovered, none of us is exempt. For some, however, the odds of joining the statistics are greater than for others.

Age

"It's a disease of working-age people," says Jerold Lancourt, M.D., an orthopedic surgeon specializing in spine rehabilitation in private practice in Dallas, "and that's why it's so disabling." Back pain can start as early as the twenties, though many patients report their troubles began between the ages

SMART DEFINITION

Orthopedics

Medical specialty devoted to the diagnosis, treatment, rehabilitation, and prevention of injuries and diseases of the musculoskeletal system, including the bones, joints, ligaments, tendons, muscles, and nerves. The word originates from the Greek words *ortho* (meaning "straight") and *paes* or *pais* ("child"), and early orthopedists were dedicated to the task of "straightening" children with spine and limb deformities. The modern orthopedist treats patients of all ages. (The modern spelling, *orthopedics,* erroneously refers to straightening the foot—from the Latin word *pedis.*)

of thirty-five and forty-five. The cause, however, tends to vary with age: Herniated disks, for instance, where the "cushions" between the bones of the spine shift position, are more common during the working years, with the age of onset spread relatively evenly from the twenties to the early forties, and gradually declining after that.

As people enter the fifties and sixties, stiffening of the spine due to the normal process of aging limits the motion that leads to much back pain, but degenerative problems such as spinal stenosis—a narrowing of the lower spinal column—become more common. Back pain in the later years is more often of the chronic type, and is less likely to be experienced as an acute attack. (More on acute and chronic pain in chapter 2.)

Occupation

Occupations at both ends of the scale—either very physically demanding or very sedentary—tend to increase the risk of back pain. Those working in jobs involving heavy manual labor take significantly more time off work because of back pain. Those whose professions involve exposure to vibrations, such as jackhammer operators, are also at increased risk for back pain. Caretakers, whether salaried or tending to elderly parents or young children at home, also run an increased risk.

According to the Department of Health and Human Services, of the 9 million working women with back pain, about one-third attributed the pain to work-related activities or injuries, with the figure rising to more than one-half among women employed in service or blue-collar occupations.

Sedentary occupations, too, add to the likelihood of back pain and herniated disks. Not only will the lack of physical activity take its toll on muscle condition, or, more accurately, the lack of it, but the very act of remaining seated for hours at a time exerts significant pressure on the back.

Posture

Different postures exert different amounts of pressure on intervertebral disks, which cushion the bones of the spine. When we are lying down, for example, disk pres-sures have been approximated at 165 pounds per square inch, compared with 220 pounds per inch while we are standing or walking, and 300 to 400 pounds while we are sitting. Not only do those who sit during a large portion of the day weaken their back muscles and the support the muscles provide, but they exert great pressure on the disk areas near the spinal cord and nerve roots, which are poorly supported areas to begin with.

Pregnancy

At least 50 percent of pregnancies involve back pain. The good news: the patient is usually freed from the pain following the delivery of her child.

Gender

Excluding the back pain related to pregnancy, there is little difference in the incidence of back pain in men and women. For all those predominately male construction workers at increased risk, there are predominately female caretakers matching them ache for ache.

Height and Weight

Tall people have been found to have a greater incidence of back pain than their shorter counter-

SMART MOVE

"Even healthy, fit people can experience back pain," says William Lauerman, M.D., associate professor of orthopedic surgery and chief of the Division of Spinal Surgery at Georgetown University Medical Center in Washington, D.C., "but the individual who weighs the appropriate amount and is in good physical condition is significantly less likely [to experience back pain] than an overweight individual who's sedentary except for going to his stressful, physically demanding job."

parts, in part due to a tendency to stoop, either to appear shorter or simply to function in a world geared to smaller-sized human beings. Also, the greater the height, the greater the weight and force the lower spine must support.

Obesity is one of the most common contributing factors to back pain. Every pound added to the "gut," one leading rehabilitation center warns its patients, adds ten pounds of pressure to the spine. The sedentary lifestyle associated with obesity and an unbalanced diet that doesn't supply adequate nutrients contribute as well.

Are You a Candidate for Back Pain?

How much at risk might you be for suffering with back ailments? The more of these questions to which you can answer yes, the more careful you should be when you bend to pick that piece of paper up off the floor, grab the baby, or reach for the phone across your desk.

1. Does your job involve heavy physical labor?

2. Are you between the ages of thirty-five and forty-five?

3. Are you overweight?

4. Do you lead a sedentary lifestyle, without regular exercise or physical activity?

5. Do you sit for great periods of time?

6. Do you smoke?

7. Are you pregnant?

8. Are you significantly taller than average?

9. Are you under stress?

10. Are you depressed?

Smoking

Odd as it might sound, back pain is yet another one of the numerous reasons to kick this habit. Significant evidence shows an increased prevalence of low-back pain associated with smoking. This might be blamed not only on related unhealthy lifestyle patterns often found among smokers but on physical reasons as well.

"Smokers cough more, and coughing increases intra-abdominal pressure, which increases pressure on the disks," says William C. Lauerman, M.D., associate professor of orthopedic surgery and chief of the Division of Spinal Surgery at Georgetown University Medical Center in Washington, D.C. "Smoking also interferes with the microcirculation to the disk, and it's well accepted that disks degenerate faster in smokers."

Add to that the fact that the worsened circulation of smokers slows healing in general. Plus, when you're experiencing back pain, coughing can make it feel all the worse.

State of Mind

Those who are under stress, depressed, or fatigued are also in the increased risk category. In such states, our coping skills are hampered, and we're less apt to guard against injury or properly care for ourselves.

"[People experiencing emotional stress] make mistakes," says orthopedist Lancourt. "It's very rare that you get in trouble when you're bright-eyed, fresh, and prepared."

In addition, the perception of physical pain can be magnified by a poor emotional state. In a vicious circle, the back pain can cause depression and withdrawal, which can overly prolong inactivity, which can decondition muscles and add extra weight, which can add back strain, and on and on.

Anatomy of the Back

Although we do not need to memorize the names and parts of the bewilderingly innumerable body components that at times seem to exist for the sole purpose of making us feel pain, understanding some basic back anatomy can provide useful insight into the way the back functions, how to keep it from malfunctioning, and how to better cope with those malfunctions if they do occur.

The Spine

The spine, or backbone, more accurately called the *spinal column* or *vertebral column,* consists of twenty-four *vertebrae* (*vertebra* in the singular form, from the Latin *vertere,* to turn). These moveable, more or less cylindrical bones are stacked one on top of another, cushioned by intervertebral disks, and connected by joints and ligaments, something we'll discuss later in this chapter.

In nearly all vertebrates—and that includes mammals, birds, reptiles, amphibians, and fishes— the spine not only provides major support to the body but protects the spinal cord, which, along with the brain, is a major component of the central nervous system (more about the spinal cord ahead). The spinal column reaches from the base of the skull to the *coccyx,* or tailbone.

No matter how much our mothers might want us to "sit up straight," our back is far more curvy than sticklike. In fact, there are three main curves to the spinal column: The two *lordotic curves* curve toward the front of the body and occur at the top of the spine (at the neck) and toward its base (beginning around the midsection, or stomach area). The curve at the neck is referred to as the *cervical lordosis;* the one that causes the hollow in the small of the back is called the *lumbar lordosis.* Between the two lordotic curves, around chest level, the *kyphotic curve* curves backward, allowing for a chest cavity and the room we need for our heart and lungs. This curve is also known as the *thoracic* or *dorsal kyphosis.*

We're not born with these curves; they develop soon afterward, and provide far greater elasticity than a straight line would allow. If their angle of curvature is too extreme or too shallow, there is more of a strain on the back and the abdominal muscles, ligaments, and tendons involved in keeping us upright.

The top seven vertebrae, located in the neck, make up the upper or cervical lordotic curve and are called the *cervical vertebrae*—in medical shorthand, C1 to C7, with C1 at the top and C7 at the bottom. Within the cervical vertebrae—which are the smallest of the vertebrae—three are of particular note: The *atlas* (C1) and the *axis* (C2) are shaped differently than the others and aren't separated by a disk. The ringlike atlas, with flat surfaces on each side, is named after the mythical Greek giant who bore the world's weight on his shoulders. It is the atlas that supports the head and allows us to nod "yes" as the skull pivots forward and back on it. Fitting into an opening in the atlas, a post protruding upward from the axis allows us to shake the head "no." The seventh cervical vertebra, the *vertebra prominens,* is characterized by a

F.Y.I.

Whether human, hamster, or giraffe, all mammals, no matter how long their necks, have seven cervical vertebrae.

prominent ridge that can be felt at the base of the neck.

The next twelve vertebrae, forming the thoracic kyphosis, are referred to as *thoracic vertebrae* (T1 to T12) or *dorsal vertebrae*. Each is attached to a pair of the ribs. The bottom five vertebrae, forming the bottom (or *lumbar*) lordotic curve, are *lumbar vertebrae* (L1 to L5), the largest vertebrae of all.

Each vertebrae has two sections: a cylinder-shaped *anterior* section called the *body* or *centrum*, facing forward; and the more irregularly shaped *posterior* section, or *arch*, toward the back. *Endplates* at the top and bottom of the anterior sections attach to the disks that separate and cushion the vertebrae. The anterior sections are the "weight-lifters"; the largest ones, down in the lumbar region, can support up to three hundred pounds per square inch. The posterior sections have somewhat spiky-looking pieces of bone interlocking with similar parts of other vertebrae to form the hollow *spinal* or *vertebral canal* for the protection of the spinal cord. The canal is largest in the areas where the spine is most flexible, such as the neck and loins, where it is wide and triangular; it is narrow and rounded toward the center of the back.

Pedicles are two short, thick pieces of bone that project backward, one on each side, from the upper part of the body of the vertebra. *Laminae* are two broad plates of bone that form the space that protects the spinal cord and are connected to the body via the pedicles.

Below the twenty-four moveable vertebrae are vertebrae that begin as individuals but end up comprising two larger anatomical bodies: the *sacrum*, at birth, is made up of five (rarely, four or six) *sacral vertebrae* that eventually fuse into one large, downward-pointing triangular bone, curved

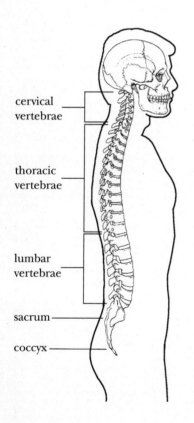

cervical vertebrae

thoracic vertebrae

lumbar vertebrae

sacrum

coccyx

and tilted in such a way as to allow room for the pelvic cavity. Early in life, the sacral vertebrae are separated from each other by disks, but by about the age of eighteen the two lowest segments become joined by ossification (the process of bone formation) extending through the disk. The process gradually continues upward until all the segments are united and the bone is completely formed by the age of twenty-five to thirty. Because the sections remain visible, they can be identified as S1 to S5. Ligaments on each side of the sacrum attach it to the *ilia,* the two large bones of the pelvis, via the *sacroiliac (SI) joints.*

Below the sacrum is the *coccyx* (from the Greek *kokkyx,* or cuckoo, for its supposed resemblance to a cuckoo's beak), which consists of four or, less often, three or five small *coccygeal vertebrae*—the topmost being the largest—that, like those of the sacrum, fuse together completely by the age of twenty-five or thirty, from the bottom vertebra up. Late in life, especially in women, the coccyx often fuses with the sacrum.

Altogether, the average spine measures about two feet three inches along the curved anterior surface of the column. The cervical region accounts for approximately five inches, the thoracic or dorsal area about eleven inches, and the lumbar vertebrae for roughly seven inches, with the sacrum and coccyx making up the remainder. Women's spines are in general about one inch shorter than men's.

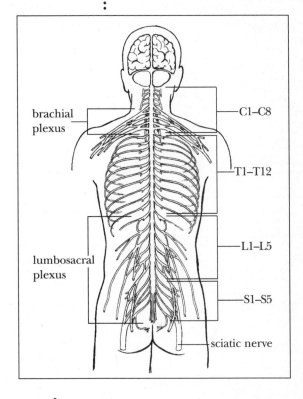

brachial plexus

C1–C8

T1–T12

L1–L5

S1–S5

lumbosacral plexus

sciatic nerve

"The first time it happened was just before my fortieth birthday," recalls Jean, of Atlanta. "I just bent over to pick something up and the pain shot through my lower back and incapacitated me. A day or two later, shooting pains began to travel down my right thigh to my toes. Until I spoke to my doctor, I was terrified that the problem was going to spread until my entire body was involved. My self-education program began that very day."

Processes, Facet Joints, and Disks

Protruding from the laminae of each vertebra, at the back section of the spinal canal, are seven features known as *processes.* Two *transverse processes* stick out sideways; and the *spinous process* points back and downward, accounting for the ridges you can feel along the spine. Both these types of processes allow for the attachment of muscles and ligaments.

It is via the four remaining processes, however, that the vertebrae "connect." At the top of each vertebra are two *superior articular processes,* and at the bottom there are two *inferior articular processes,* with each of the four articular processes having a smooth *facet* at its end. The two superior articular processes of each vertebra join with the two inferior articular processes of the vertebra above it at the *facet joint,* encased in a *joint capsule* that keeps the facets from coming apart at the same time as it allows them to move about. Cartilage capping the facets provides for smooth movement rather than friction.

Acting like shock absorbers and keeping bones from grinding against each other, *intervertebral disks* separate the mobile vertebrae (with the exception of the atlas and axis), buffering them against jarring and injury. The disks themselves account for about 25 percent of the spine's length; stacked one atop the other, they'd reach about six inches in height. Disks in different parts of the spine vary in shape (oval in the cervical and lumbar regions; circular in the thoracic or dorsal) and size (largest and thickest in the lumbar region). Proportionally, the thoracic or dorsal portion of the spine has a much smaller quantity of intervertebral material than do the cervical and lumbar regions, giving the latter parts greater flexibility and freedom of movement.

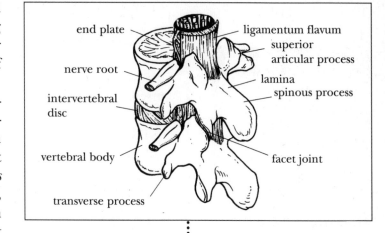

Each disk has two sections. The tough, protective, fibrous outer section is the *annulus fibrosus.* At its center is the *nucleus pulposus,* a soft, elastic, pulpy mass, yellowish in color, that is gelatinous at infancy and becomes increasingly less fluid and more sinewy as our bodies age. When functioning properly, the nucleus pulposus changes shape water-balloon-like to accommodate our movement before reverting to its initial form.

At birth, each nucleus is made of approximately 90 percent water. The percentage slowly decreases until, by the time we're in our seventies, it's declined to about 70 percent. But far from a strictly one-way process, disks' absorption and loss of water occurs on a daily basis. During waking hours, the force of gravity on our bodies causes water to leave the disks' centers, and they flatten out a bit. During sleep, the water content is replenished, soaking into the disks via the circulatory system, which also provides nutrients. That's why most of us are a little bit taller when we awaken than when we go to bed, and why astronauts spending extended periods of time in the weightlessness of space return to earth inches taller (at least temporarily) than when they'd left.

Disks are identified by the vertebrae they cushion. The disk between the third and fourth cervical vertebrae is called C3-C4, or C3-4; that between the bottom lumbar vertebra and the sacrum would be L5-S1.

Ligaments and Muscles

Ligaments are the tough bands of tissue that connect one bone to another. They support the spine and prevent us from moving in ways that might result in our hurting ourselves.

The *ligamenta subflava* (whose yellow color has earned it the nickname "the yellow ligament") connects the laminae; and the *capsular, supraspinous, interspinous,* and *intertransverse ligaments* connect the processes. Two *longitudinal ligaments*—the *anterior* longitudinal ligament attached to the front section of the vertebral bodies and disks, and the *posterior* longitudinal ligament attached to the back—run the length of the spinal column.

Muscles are very elastic tissues that, by expanding and contracting, allow the body to move, and, while they're at it, support the skeletal structure. In total, there are fifty-six muscles directly attached to the vertebrae (twenty pair to the atlas and axis alone). Although the muscles of the back are generally thought of in five layers, for simplicity's sake we'll discuss them on three basic levels: Farthest from the surface are very short muscles allowing delicate movements, bends, and twists within the bounds set by the ligaments. Other short muscles are attached to the facet joints which, depending on their structure, will move forward, backward, sideways, or rotate to different degrees.

The next level of muscles are longer, extending from vertebra to vertebra. Above these is the *erector spinae* or *sacrospinalis*, a group of long muscles that extend the length of the spine. When they are contracted, the spine arches back. When the muscles on one side are tightened, the spine bends sideways. The erector spinae also brace the spine from the rear, holding the body upright. Of the relatively few muscles attached to the front of the vertebrae are the *major* and *minor psoas muscles,* with the main functions of flexing the thigh, trunk, and the lumbar spine.

The ability to bend forward—and not fall over backward when we stand—depends not on back muscles, but on abdominal muscles. The deepest layer, comprised of the *obliquus internis* and the *obliquus externis* (also known as the *internal and external obliques*) reaches diagonally from hip bones to ribs. Next, the *transversus abdominis* crosses the lower layer. Above that, the *rectus abdominis* runs vertically. When all are contracted, the spine bends forward. When those on one side are contracted, the spine bends to the side.

Strong abdominal muscles are also important. When the erector spinae and abdominal muscles are comparable in strength, they work together to help your body maintain an erect posture without too much strain. When the abdominal muscles are weak, it puts more of a burden on the spine, leaving it more vulnerable to wear and tear and injury.

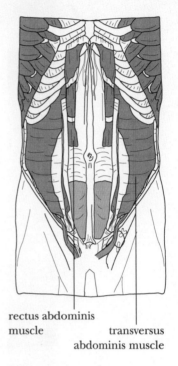

rectus abdominis
muscle

transversus
abdominis muscle

Spinal Cord and Nerves

Among the most complex parts of the back is the *spinal cord* (*medulla spinalis*), which, together with the brain, forms the central nervous system. The central nervous system, in turn, supervises and coordinates the activity of the entire nervous system, which basically tells our bodies what they need to do to survive. No small feat.

F.Y.I.

Although many nerve endings are sensitive to pain, not all are. The nerves to the nuclei of the disks and the muscles, for instance, do not contain pain receptors.

For all its weighty function, the spinal cord itself—without its membranes or nerves—weighs about an ounce and a half. It runs from the base of the brain down through the spinal canal, and, within the canal, is protected by layers of fibrous tissue: going from innermost to outermost, the *pia mater,* the *arachnoid,* and the *dura mater.*

During the embryonic stages of life, the spinal cord extends from the brain to the sacrum, but, because the vertebrae "outgrow" it, by the time we're born, the spinal cord merely reaches L3, the third lumbar vertebra. In the adult, it's about seventeen to eighteen inches in length, and occupies the upper two-thirds of the vertebral canal, with the end of the spinal cord (the *conus medullaris*) extending only as far as L1.

From the spinal cord branches a system of thousands of *nerves,* which deliver and receive messages—sensation and all manner of information—to and from every part of the body. The nerves develop from sixty-two main branches called *nerve roots,* each of which emerges from the spinal column—thirty-one on each side of the column—through an intervertebral space before branching off into nerves.

Branches of the nerve roots from the neck, or cervical area, handle messages to and from the upper areas of the body, such as the arms and shoulders. Branches of the nerve roots from the lumbar region relate to the lower areas of the body, such as the legs and feet.

The *sciatic nerve,* for instance, the thickest nerve in the body, measuring three-quarters of an inch in breadth, runs down the back of each thigh, splits into two branches above the knee, and continues: one branch down the front of the shin to the big toe; the other branch down the back of the leg to the heel and the front of the leg to the other toes. Strands of nerves, like the sciatic, that exit below L1, where the spinal cord ends, are called the *cauda equina* (Latin for "horse's tail").

Back Pain in the Leg?

You're feeling shooting pains in your calf, and you didn't even go jogging. Your shoulder is killing you and you haven't a clue as to the cause—probably because you're looking in the wrong place.

Referred pain, the appearance of pain in an area other than its cause, is not unusual when it comes to the back, where so many nerves originate before branching to other parts of the body. Symptoms of spinal stenosis, for instance, a narrowing of the spinal canal, can include aches in the buttock, thigh, and calf. A bulging disk pressing on a nerve in the lower back region can cause shooting pain, weakness, or numbness in the legs; a pinched nerve in the neck can be felt in the shoulders and arms.

"The nerve is pinched in the back but that nerve's job is to provide function and feeling to, say, the leg," explains surgeon Jerold Lancourt. "So that nerve can't say, 'I'm being pinched in the back.' The nerve's function is all centered on the leg, so no matter where it's injured it's going to say 'Ouch!' in the area that it serves. In low back pain, it goes down the leg, in rare thoracic [mid-back] problems it goes around the chest or abdomen, and in neck pain it goes down the arms, depending on which nerves are involved."

"There are two ways that a patient can experience referred pain," elaborates William Lauerman of Georgetown University Medical Center. "One is

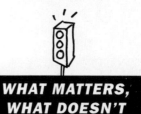

WHAT MATTERS, WHAT DOESN'T

What Matters

• Knowing the risk factors for back pain and reducing or eliminating those we can.

• Understanding that the parts of the back connect with other parts of the body.

• Recognizing that back pain prevention requires taking care of *all* the back's parts as well as the adbomen.

What Doesn't

• Knowing the names of each and every part of the back.

• That your "back pain" occurs in places other than your back. It can still originate there.

• Having strong back muscles that aren't complemented by strong abdominal muscles.

truly referred pain, meaning that tissue at one site is injured or irritated and causes pain to be perceived in another site." An example of this is the buttock or leg pain caused by a degenerated disk in the lower spine.

"Another way that a patient can experience pain like this is *radicular pain,*" says Lauerman. One source of radicular pain is spinal stenosis, mentioned earlier, where narrowing of the spinal canal either from arthritis and overgrowth of the joints, a herniated disk, or congenital factors squeezes the spinal nerves, leading to pain, numbness, or tingling that radiates down into the buttock, thigh, or even down the leg. Both types of pain can occur at the same time.

"With true referred pain, people usually feel pain in or around the midline of their back, enough to recognize that it may well be a back problem," says Lauerman. "With radicular pain, it's not uncommon for someone to think they have a pulled hamstring or a pinched nerve in their leg or even their foot because the symptoms all seem to be concentrated there. It's the exception rather than the rule, but certainly occurs in a significant number of people."

Conversely, pains in the back are sometimes due to ailments in other parts of the body. Among the most common nonorthopaedic causes are pancreatitis, kidney stones, peptic ulcers, abdominal aortic aneurysms, or maladies of the ovaries, fallopian tubes, or uterus. Prostate or other cancers elsewhere in the body can also be to blame.

No wonder we cannot always diagnose our own back problems. In the next chapter we look at how health professionals find out what's wrong, and we discuss the most common causes.

THE BOTTOM LINE

Although back pain can strike anyone, many problems can be prevented by replacing bad habits with better ones—and the sooner, the better. Even when we are already aching, there are steps we can take to reduce recovery time and, afterward, make that recovery more lasting. Familiarity with our anatomy can help us along, and understanding back pain's ability to appear in other parts of the body can help hasten diagnosis.

Back Pain, Specialists, and Tests

THE KEYS

• Knowing the exact cause or source of back pain isn't crucial to getting relief.

• Although most back pain will heal itself, there are times when a visit to the doctor is advisable, and other times when it's a must.

• From conservative to holistic, different medical specialties offer a variety of different approaches to diagnosis and treatment.

• A wide range of diagnostic tests provides an in-depth view of the back and what might be causing its problems.

In the last chapter we learned that back pain sufferers are members of an enormous, if reluctant, club of people of every age, gender, profession, color, and creed. If a back pain experience can be considered a club meeting, a rare few of us attend just once in our lives; most of us meet on an irregular but recurrent basis; and a few of us live in the clubhouse full-time.

A look at the anatomical components that comprise the back was our first step in learning what can go wrong to cause pain and understanding why the pain can't even be counted upon to confine itself to the part of our bodies in which it originates. In this chapter we'll take a brief look at some of the more common, if elusive, causes of back pain and explore some of the ways in which health care professionals try to track it down.

Common Causes of Pain: The Short Answer

If you are the kind of person who cannot rest without knowing the answer, prepare for a long, sleepless night. Even with all the wonders of modern medical technology, the exact reason for or cause of back pain most often goes undetected. In a large majority of cases it falls into the category of what's called nonspecified back pain, which, happily, heals itself although an anatomical explanation may never be found.

Let's briefly review the anatomy lesson in chapter 1: The spine is made up of bones called *verte-*

brae, stacked atop each other to form a column, with cushioning *disks* between them. *Ligaments* hold the vertebrae together, and *muscles,* allowing movement, are attached to the vertebrae by bands of tissue called *tendons.* Openings in the vertebrae line up to form a long hollow canal that houses the *spinal cord,* which runs from the base of the brain to about two-thirds of the way down the spine. *Nerves* branch out from the spinal cord, emerging from spaces between the vertebrae.

The pain can hide in any one of these many parts. And more. That's a lot of parts. And, just as bones, muscles, ligaments, and tendons are interconnected to help each other, a problem in one area can cause pain in another.

In most events, it is believed that the anguish originates in weakness in or damage to the spine's many support structures—muscles, ligaments, and joints—which, once they are compromised, can weaken or result in damage to other structures, including disks, nerves, and the vertebrae themselves. The initial weakness or damage can itself be blamed on everything from a sedentary lifestyle to poor posture or nutrition to the aging process to disease. In turn, any or all of these factors and others can leave us more susceptible to physical injury, another common cause of pain.

According to the Back Association of Canada (BAC), a Toronto-based foundation established by a group of back pain sufferers and health care professionals, finding an effective program of back pain treatment in most cases calls only for knowledge of the general category (or categories) of problem to be known. "Narrowing the problem down further doesn't usually make a whole lot of difference since the conservative treatment for each category is more or less the same," according

SMART DEFINITION

Pain

An unpleasant sensory and emotional experience associated with actual or potential tissue damage, or described in terms of such damage.

Source: International Association for the Study of Pain

SMART SOURCES

Back Association of
 Canada
83 Cottingham St.
Toronto, Ontario
Canada M4V 1B9
416-967-4670
www.backassociation.ca

This nonprofit founda-
tion established by a
group of back pain
sufferers and health
care professionals
offers a range of fun-
to-read and easily
understood information
on diagnosis and treat-
ment. Its main goal:
educating back pain
sufferers in order to
help them make wiser
personal decisions. A
voluntary membership
donation covers all
educational materials
BAC produces during
the year, as well as
free copies of several
informational bro-
chures, published in
English and French.
Founder Judylaine
Fine's *The Ultimate
Back Book* is a great
source of valuable
information.

to BAC's Web site, which lists the five main causes of pain as:

1. Sprains and strains of the muscles, ligaments, and tendons

2. Disk problems

3. Facet joint problems

4. Osteoarthritis (also called degenerative arthritis, or degenerative joint disease, because it's related to age-related changes in the bones and joints)

5. Spinal stenosis, a narrowing of the spinal canal that can develop because of a congenital defect or as a result of osteoarthritis.

We'll look more closely into these categories and specific maladies in chapter 3. First, we'll examine the methods of examination, and the kinds of health care professionals who conduct them.

Chronic or Acute?

Not only can it be difficult to tell where the back pain is coming from—it can even be hard to tell whether the pain is acute or chronic, and that can affect treatment.

In general, *acute pain* is the initial pain people feel after an injury. In most cases, the body will begin healing itself, and the patient's job is simply to relieve the pain and keep the injured area safe un-

til fully recovered. If the pain lasts longer than expected—which, for back pain, is usually considered
to be about six weeks at most—or is due to an ongoing condition such as arthritis, the pain is considered *chronic,* and a different treatment plan
comes into play.

Although chronic back pain is, in most cases,
not directly caused by injury, the source of the pain
can bring about an injury that then appears to be
the culprit. For instance, poor muscle tone de-
prives the spine of necessary support, puts stress
upon the joints, and leaves the back more susceptible to injury.

Some schools of thought hold that chronic
pain is the end of a chain of nervous system events
that starts in the brain and ends with pain in the
back. In its most basic form, for instance, emotional stress can lead to physical muscle tension,
which can lead to pain (and injury, which, in our
stressed state, we're more likely to become victim
to). Because the nervous system is connected to
the mind and the emotions, the theory goes, healing is best directed there. See chapter 7 for more
about the mind-body connection.

Categorizing your pain as acute or chronic can
be a subjective call. Are those intermittent
episodes of acute pain you're experiencing, or is it
a series of recurrent episodes stemming from the
same source? Does the pain never seem to leave,
becoming only relatively better and worse?

Dos and Don'ts for
Acute and Chronic Back Pain

The best treatment for the pain that arises after a full day at work in the garden might not be appropriate for an ache that's been bothering you for several weeks.

Acute

• **Apply ice now.** Apply a cold pack or ice to the area within the first forty-eight hours (the sooner, the better), for no longer than five to ten minutes at a time, allowing twenty minutes between applications.

• **Apply heat later.** If symptoms last longer than two days, heat (heating pad, hot shower, or bath) might help relieve symptoms.

• **Consider the laying on of hands.** Spinal manipulation by a trained health care professional such as a physical therapist or chiropractor can help during the first month. If symptoms continue, see a medical doctor.

Acute and Chronic

• **Learn to relax.** Taking it easy physically *and* mentally will ease muscle tension.

• **Rest, but don't overdo it.** Like emotional stress, long periods of inactivity can make back symptoms seem worse and work against physical recovery.

• **Act sensibly.** Learn and take part in an appropriate exercise routine to strengthen your back and supporting muscles and improve flexibility.

• **Take it easy.** Especially when pain is severe, avoid heavy lifting; lifting when twisting, bending forward, and reaching; and standing or sitting for long periods of time.

• **Do tell.** Let your family and co-workers know if your pain interferes with your normal daily activities, and don't attempt any "heroics" that might make it worse.

• **Get help.** If the pain is long-lasting, a doctor's visit is due.

When to See a Doctor and What Type of Doctor to See

"When you have excruciating pain that you just can't tolerate, that's almost always time to see the doctor," says Garth S. Russell, M.D., an orthopedic surgeon in Palm Beach Gardens, Florida. "But usually back pain comes from an acute strain, which will last moderately severely for about two days and then will gradually improve over the next two weeks, so that all a person has to do is to rest until the acute pain subsides and then just gradually increase their activity, and the pain will go away."

As another orthopedic surgeon put it: "Most back pain is a self-limited disease. Duck and get out of the way, and Mother Nature will cure you if you leave it alone."

A visit to the doctor is advisable in some cases, however, such as when there are signs of neurological (nerve-related) trouble—for example, weakness in the legs, or loss of bowel or bladder function.

"That does not necessarily mean surgery," Dr. Russell notes, "but these patients need to get to a doctor and get a little more supervised treatment. The doctor will examine them and if he finds that the nerves are pressured but are still functioning, he has time to treat them conservatively." Gentle physical therapy, a course of moderate exercise, mild pain medication, muscle relaxants, or a short-term course of steroids or cortisone might be prescribed to relieve the pain.

As for the type of doctor to see, there are almost as many choices as there are vertebrae. In addition to the basic family practitioner (known in this HMO era as the primary care physician), who sees most of us when our back pain sends us physician-ward, there are orthopedic surgeons, neurosurgeons, physiatrists, rheumatologists, neurologists, and radiologists; not to mention physical therapists, chiropractors, osteopaths, massage therapists, and a host of other health care professionals.

One of the keys to treatment success by any of these trained healers is that his or her treatment philosophy is compatible with yours. In other words: Do you trust him? Are you confident of her credentials? Enough people are turning to chiropractors so as to challenge the use of the word "alternative" in connection with the therapy. Others are open to considering the help of acupuncturists or massage therapists and learning yoga or bodywork techniques (see chapter 7 for these and other such approaches). Whatever else is uncertain about back pain, you certainly won't want for willing help.

See the Doctor If . . .

• You develop numbness or weakness in the legs.

• Symptoms are extremely severe or disabling and do not subside within several days.

• Pain lasts more than six to eight weeks.

• Pain is accompanied by fever and/or unexplained weight loss.

• Pain recurs more than twice a year.

See the Doctor Right Away If . . .

• You lose bowel or bladder control.

• You experience numbness in the groin or rectal area.

• You experience extreme leg weakness or pain extending below the knee accompanied by a tingling or "pins and needles" sensation.

The Unexpected Specialists

Orthopedics, which was defined briefly in chapter 1, is likely the first medical specialty to come to mind when we think of the back. The back, after all, brings to mind the spine, which brings to mind the bones, and for informed readers like you, the muscles, joints, ligaments, tendons, and other components of the musculoskeletal system, which is the area of specialty of the orthopedic surgeon. Meanwhile, it turns out that two of the most frequently referred specialists—neurosurgeons and physiatrists—play a vital role.

Neurosurgeons

Patients with back pain symptoms that include weakness in the foot or other signs of a neurologic deficit will most often be referred to a neurosurgeon or neurological surgeon, who is, in the simplest terms, a medical specialist whose focus is on your nerves.

F.Y.I.

In the United States:

Board certified
neurosurgeons: 4,599[*]

Board certified
physiatrists   5,886[†]

Board certified
orthopedic
surgeons: 22,127[‡]

[*] American Board of Neurological Surgery
[†] American Board of Physical Medicine and Rehabilitation
[‡] American Board of Orthopaedic Surgery

SMART MOVE

Whatever variety of qualified back care professional you see, don't hesitate to see another to confirm his or her diagnosis. "A good person who's giving good advice is not afraid of a second opinion and won't punish you as a patient," says Richard Toselli, M.D., director of the Spine Center at the University of North Carolina at Chapel Hill. "Patients get the feeling sometimes that some doctors are not receptive to that. If they're not, then maybe you need to find somebody else."

It may come as a surprise to learn that the health care professionals so often thought of as brain surgeons more often deal with the back. Sixty percent of the members of the American Association of Neurological Surgeons (AANS), the largest neurosurgical organization in North America, in fact, say they are exclusively spine surgeons, according to spokesperson Susan A. Nowicki. And lumbar/thoracic spine problems are the most common condition these medical specialists see.

The neurosurgeon is not just there to operate, but provides either surgical or nonsurgical care, depending on the nature of the injury or illness.

"Education is the biggest thing a neurosurgeon does," says Richard M. Toselli, M.D., clinical associate professor of neurosurgery and director of the Spine Center at the University of North Carolina at Chapel Hill. "We spend a lot of our day keeping people from surgery," he adds. "It's not just a doctor problem, it's a patient perception. People need to understand that if they hurt it doesn't always mean that they need an operation when it comes to the spine."

Neurosurgeons have extensive training in the diagnosis and treatment of patients with injury to, or diseases of, the brain, spine, or peripheral nerves (nerves dealing with the face, arms, legs, hands, and feet), but, as mentioned earlier, many specialize in or confine their practice to the back.

Like an orthopedic surgeon, the neurosurgeon might be the only doctor you see after referral—or he or she might be consulted by or be part of a team including primary care practitioners, physiatrists, and others.

A neurologist is yet another professional who is skilled in the diagnosis and treatment of problems related to the nervous system, but does not perform surgery.

The Spinal Cord and Nervous System

One of the crucial functions of the spinal column is to protect the spinal cord, which can be thought of as an extension of the brain. All the information going from the brain to the limbs, allowing our bodies to move, goes through the spinal cord. It's been called "the first relay station" for sensory information on its way to the different parts of the brain. Bladder functions, sensory functions, and movement all depend on information traveling up and down the spinal cord.

Physiatrists

Nothing Freudian about them, physiatrists (the word is pronounced *fizzy-AT-rists*) focus on the diagnosis and treatment of physical disability. Physiatrists (from the Greek *physikos* for physical, and *iatreia,* the art of healing) are also known as specialists in the field of physical medicine and rehabilitation. Patients are often referred to a physiatrist by the primary care physician.

Physiatry was recognized as a medical specialty in 1947, with the goal of helping the physically disabled reach their maximum potential. One nationwide study done in the mid-1980s of five hundred sufferers of neck and low back pain pronounced physiatrists the "best bet" among practitioners.

Like other back care specialists, physiatrists can help patients with a wide range of ills, acute and chronic, and can address neurologic and orthopedic complaints. What sets them apart from other health care professionals is a specialization in whole-person health, including the physical, emotional, and social components of a healthy, func-

SMART SOURCES

American Academy of
  Physical Medicine
  and Rehabilitation
One IBM Plaza,
  Suite 2500
Chicago, IL 60611
312-464-9700
www.aapmr.org

Representing physiatrists throughout the United States and Canada, AAPM&R provides the public with a wealth of information about the medical specialty as well as referrals to board-certified practitioners.

tional life. Unlike other medical professionals, the physiatrist isn't dealing with a threat to life, but with the quality of life. "Who should see a physiatrist? Someone whose function is less than what they wish it to be," sums up one renowned member of the field.

"This is a field to help people regain optimal function," says Stanley A. Herring, M.D., of Puget Sound Sports and Spine Physicians, who is also a clinical professor of physical medicine and rehabilitation at the University of Washington. "The difference is the emphasis on restoration of function and optimizing performance, not just relieving pain."

A holistic approach can be recognized in the taking of the patient's medical history, which might include questions of a social, emotional, and spiritual nature in addition to the usual queries about age, height, and weight. Everything from sleep behavior to the ability to get dressed to performance on the job will be assessed to provide an overall image of how the patient as a human being—not just the back of one—functions day to day. "Can you take care of your household?" "Are you having any problems at work?" "How is your home life?" "Do you find yourself feeling helpless?" These are some of the questions a physiatrist might ask.

For the physical exam, you might be asked to walk down a hallway or up and down stairs, to get into and out of a chair—perhaps ten times in a row, if repetitive movement is part of what makes up your day.

Reflecting this broad-based approach to healing, physiatrists often work with a wide variety of other health professionals to develop a rehabilitation plan. Doctors and nurses from specialties including neurology and orthopedics; physical, occupational, and/or speech therapy; psychology; vocational counseling or social work; acupuncture, chiropractic, and massage therapy might be on the team.

"When it comes to back pain, there are all kinds of opinions and belief systems, and very rarely does one person have the right approach for all patients. You really need someone to be a quarterback and an advocate," says Dr. Herring, who, as a physician for the Seattle Seahawks football team, knows the importance of teamwork.

"We take a disease and look at what types of impairment and disability are associated with it, and

A Multidisciplinary Approach

At the Spine Center at the University of North Carolina at Chapel Hill, a staff of orthopedic surgeons, neurosurgeons, physiatrists, anesthesiologists, specialists in pain management, and other health care practitioners works together to help patients whose complaints range from "I hurt my back putting in this year's tulip bulbs," to "I've had chronic back pain for years," to patients with severe spinal cord injury.

At or in close proximity to Puget Sound Sports and Spine Physicians in Seattle are two spine surgeons, a psychologist specializing in the effects of pain on mood and function, a physician who is board certified in pain management, a physical therapist, and an occupational therapist.

If we're fortunate, such clinics could be the wave of the future. More and more often, multidisciplinary programs such as these, with physicians organized by field of concern rather than by specialty of approach, are allowing the emphasis to remain on healing and relieving spinal disease and *all* of its symptoms rather than on methods of diagnosis and treatment that isolate only one part of what is usually a complex problem. With a variety of physicians joining as colleagues to treat patients in the most appropriate way, patients are more likely to be treated in the best way.

put together a plan that not only addresses symptoms but restoration," says Dr. Herring. "I cannot fix you. You have to participate. If you think I'm going to save you, you're in the wrong office."

The Clinical Exam

During your initial office visit to any doctor, expect a lot of talking. He or she will take a detailed medical history and ask a series of questions about your symptoms and what they keep you from doing. The more questions the doctor asks, and the more accurate your answers, the better for your potential working relationship.

Next is a physical exam to try to narrow down the type of pain and its cause, much of which might be guided by your answers to the questions asked during the medical history portion of the visit. Be prepared to go through a series of motions—sitting, standing, walking, and lying down in a variety of positions—that will demonstrate your range of movement, what hurts, whether there are any areas of weakness, how your reflexes are working, and how you move.

Pain related to disk problems (called diskogenic pain), for instance, tends to be worse when you put your back into a position called flexion, such as when you lean forward to touch your toes from a standing position. Returning to the upright posture will hurt less than bending over. Pain due to facet joint problems, on the other hand, might be most noticeable when the spine is in the opposite position, or extended, and will be localized to the area of the irritated joint.

Your Doctor Might Ask . . .

Communication with your health care provider is essential for ensuring the quality of your treatment. At your exam, these are some of the questions your doctor may ask. Noting your answers in advance on a sheet of paper that you take with you can be helpful during your initial exam. Answer honestly and fully.

• When did your back symptoms start?

• Which of your daily activities are you not able to do because of your back symptoms?

• Is there anything you do that makes the symptoms better or worse?

• Have you noticed any problem with your legs?

• Around the time your symptoms began, did you have a fever or symptoms of pain or burning when urinating?

• Have you had a problem with your back in the past? If so, when?

• What medical illnesses have you had (for example, cancer, arthritis, or diseases of the immune system)?

• Which medicines do you take regularly?

• Have you ever used intravenous (IV) drugs?

• Have you recently lost weight without trying?

You should also tell your health care provider about anything you may be doing for your symptoms: medicines you are taking, creams or ointments you are using, and other home remedies. Stress, depression, or substance use problems can slow recovery or make back symptoms seem worse. Tell your doctor if any of these apply to you.

Source: "Understanding Acute Low Back Problems," U.S. Department of Health and Human Services, Agency for Human Care Policy and Research.

SMART DEFINITION

Flexion
Bending forward

Extension
Bending backward

Rotation
Twisting

There are tests with nasty-sounding names like the posterior pelvic pain provocation test; and the ventral and dorsal gapping tests, and those that are friendlier sounding, such as Patrick's test to evaluate the sacroiliac area. For the valsalva maneuver, the patient holds his breath and strains as if for a bowel movement; pain traveling down the leg might indicate disk herniation.

The Diagnostic Dilemma

In most cases of physical illness or disability, the general rule is that without a specific diagnosis of where the pain is coming from, or what is its cause, there is little chance of treating that pain or hastening recovery. When it comes to most back pain, however, no such rule applies.

It's much more important to see which patient has the disease than which disease the patient has, to paraphrase the renowned Canadian physician and medical historian Sir William Osler. For back pain patients, the statement is particularly true. Muscle strain, bone spurs, even pinched nerves can mean significantly different things to different people.

"Symptoms and pathology do not always correlate in back pain," says physiatrist Stanley Herring, on the board of directors of the North American Spine Society. Indeed, a study reported in the *New England Journal of Medicine* found that of ninety-eight people *without* back pain, almost two-thirds were shown to have one or more herniated disks or other spinal abnormality when scanned by a technique called magnetic resonance imaging or MRI. "You don't treat the MRI," notes Dr. Herring. "You treat the patient."

Irregularities in an MRI do not always mean injury; because they don't show cause, tests can reveal abnormalities with which you were born, but that have nothing to do with your present pain.

Nevertheless, a lot of MRIs, and many other diagnostic tests, are being performed. In 1993, the North Carolina Back Pain Project examined the patterns of diagnostic test use among primary care physicians and the specialty practices of orthopedic surgeons and chiropractors. Researchers found the availability of both basic diagnostic technology (such as X-rays), and of sophisticated imaging tests (such as computerized tomography and MRIs) "has broadened in recent years," and, along with it, so have doctors' tendencies to use them. According to the study, "the use of imaging for diagnosis appeared to occur too early and too frequently."

Since then, the pendulum seems to have started toward the other direction. "I think there has over the past five years or so been some movement for physicians to become more conservative in utilization of diagnostic tests," says Timothy S. Carey, M.D., M.P.H., professor of medicine at the University of North Carolina at Chapel Hill, who coauthored the study. "Especially early in the back pain."

This isn't the only study that supports federal Agency for Health Care Policy and Research (AHCPR) guidelines in recommending a conservative approach to diagnostic testing. In its controversial report, accused by some of being more cost-conscious than patient-conscious, the AHCPR divided acute back pain into "red flag" pain that needs a lot of care and investigation; and the pain that needs supportive treatment but will get better

SMART SOURCES

"Understanding Acute Low Back Problems" is a free brochure produced by the U.S. Department of Health and Human Services' Agency for Health Care Policy and Research. To order, call 800-358-9295; write to the Publications Clearinghouse, P.O. Box 8547, Silver Spring, MD 20907; or, to have the pamphlet faxed to you right away, contact AHCPR's around-the-clock InstantFAX line: dial 301-594-2800 from your fax machine handset and request document number 950644.

no matter what you do. Red-flag patients might include those who have had serious trauma, such as a fall from a ladder, and require X-rays to rule out fracture; patients with a history of infection, which is a rare cause of back pain; patients with a history of malignant cancer; those with weakened bones from steroids or osteoporosis; and patients who have been in pain for an extended period of time, generally thought to be more than four to six weeks. Worsening neurological findings (say, numbness in the foot on Monday, and weakness in the foot on Tuesday) would also be among the red flags.

In most other cases, "little is lost by delaying diagnostic testing for several weeks to determine whether spontaneous recovery will occur," concurs the North Carolina Back Pain Project study.

"Over 90 percent will be better prior to six weeks on their own," says Dr. Carey, adding, "While the good news is chances are it's going to get better, the fact that it has a good prognosis doesn't make it hurt any less."

Do You Need to Get a Test?

Factors that go into deciding whether you'll be tested might include your age, how long you've been in pain, the number of previous episodes of back pain you've had, the severity of the pain, and its effect on your day-to-day functioning; it can even be influenced by the practitioner's specialty and size of practice. Dr. Carey found that, for instance, compared to primary care physicians, chiropractors and orthopedic surgeons were much more likely to take X-rays no matter how the clinical exam went.

Patient anxiety also plays a large role. With the levels of severity that back pain can reach, many request diagnostic tests for reassurance that they are not seriously hurt. That can backfire when irrelevant test results cause undue worry.

"You may see tests used to reassure the patient," says Dr. Carey, "but the problem with that is that many individuals will have variations in their spinal anatomy. Bone spurs, for instance, will be found equally in people with and without back pain." (See the *New England Journal of Medicine* study mentioned on page 34.)

"It's very frightening for people," says neurosurgeon Dr. Richard Toselli, who remembers his own bout with back pain as "the worst pain I've ever felt." "Even for me, and others in the profession, there is the question, 'Am I going to get better or did I just do something really bad?'

"Patients many times come to you with that issue: 'I hurt. I want a reason.' And if you don't have a good education component, they may be upset when they leave if you don't do a study. One of the problems is they may not *need* a study."

Diagnostic Tests for Back Pain

If your physician determines that the clinical examination has turned up something that merits confirmation or a closer look, he can choose from a wide range of diagnostic tests to be used individually or in combination with others. Many are noninvasive, meaning they do not involve needles or any other intrusion into your body, and they pre-

SMART MOVE

One "ouch" from the patient, one answer on a questionnaire, or one diagnostic test isn't enough for a doctor to plan a course of action. "One has to be very careful to put the whole picture together," says physiatrist Richard S. Materson, M.D., a professor at Baylor College of Medicine and University of Texas Health Science Center, and former president of the American Academy of Physical Medicine and Rehabilitation. "The experienced physician doesn't rely on one study or another study alone, but takes into account the whole mosaic—the history, the physical examination, the lab studies, the imaging studies and whatever tests— and they have to fit into a reliable pattern before you take any kind of action."

F.Y.I.

Percent of patients to receive an X-ray by:

Primary care providers:
  20 percent

Chiropractors:
  62 percent

Orthopedic surgeons:
  70 percent

Source: "Patterns of Ordering Diagnostic Tests for Patients with Acute Low Back Pain," *Annals of Internal Medicine,* November 15, 1996. Timothy S. Carey, M.D., M.P.H.; Joanne Garrett, Ph.D.; and the North Carolina Back Pain Project.

sent only a minimum of discomfort in exchange for the information they provide. Most are avoidable unless your doctor is convinced that the potential findings would lead to a different treatment strategy.

Most Common Diagnostic Tests

The following are the most common diagnostic tests prescribed.

Radiography or X-Rays

X-ray images—more commonly called X-rays—are produced by a form of radiation that is capable of penetrating the body and are the most commonly used method for taking an image of what's deep inside without invasive technique. Following clinical examination into the cause of your back pain, your doctor might use "plain" X-rays (see CT scans, below, for a fancier version) to look for fractures and tumors. Not great for viewing soft tissue such as disks, they can reveal bone spurs that might be pinching a nerve, as well as osteoporosis. Also known as radiographs, X-ray images are analyzed by radiographers, who are experts at deciphering what only appear as shadows to the untrained eye. Myelograms, CT scans, and other diagnostic tests (see below) involve X-rays. Continuous X-ray images can be seen through an instrument known as a fluoroscope.

Myelogram

If the clinical examination indicates you might be experiencing a pinched nerve, spinal stenosis, or some other condition your doctor believes might require surgery to remedy, a myelogram might be ordered. Although this is an invasive test that can be uncomfortable, it provides a very clear image and can reveal the extent, location, and nature of the trouble.

For the myelogram, radiopaque dye, which shows up on X-rays, is injected into the spinal canal by means of a lumbar puncture. (This same procedure is known as a spinal tap, particularly when it is used to withdraw, or "tap," spinal fluid for testing. See *cerebrospinal fluid analysis*, on page 44.) Next, the patient lies face-down on a table that is slowly tilted back and forth to allow the dye to flow through the spinal canal, outlining the spinal cord and nerve roots in the areas being studied. X-rays are taken from different angles. If dye isn't visible in a specific area, it might indicate the spinal cord or nerve root is being pinched by a herniated disk or bone spur; or the presence of scar tissue, a tumor, or cyst.

Myelograms are often done in conjunction with CT scans (see below) because the radiopaque dye produces a sharper CT scan image.

Computerized Tomography (CT) Scan

Also called a CAT (*computed axial tomography* or *computer aided tomography*) scan, the CT scan, like the myelogram, is used to confirm a clinical diagnosis of operable trouble and help pinpoint its location. Often done in conjunction with a myelogram, because the dye used in myelograms results in a clearer image, CT scans are particularly useful for providing pictures of the bony parts of the back.

SMART MOVE

You have the right to know your doctor's reasons for performing any and all diagnostic tests, and in the case of those that are invasive or expose you to radiation there's especially good cause to be informed. Timothy Carey, M.D., M.P.H., professor of medicine at the University of North Carolina at Chapel Hill, encourages you to speak up. "When a doctor says to a patient he's going to take X-rays, for example, the patient should ask, 'Why are you taking them, and how is your treatment going to be different depending on what those films show?'"

If he or she can't answer, or replies, "I get X-rays on all my patients," find another doctor.

Lying face up on a narrow, adjustable bed, the patient is slowly propelled through the "hole" of a doughnut-shaped scanner ring as the computer-controlled scanner revolves around the ring. Hundreds of thousands of scans are taken of thin transaxial slices of the spine, which are then translated by a computer into images. The result are cross-sectional views of areas as thin as one-fifth of an inch. The procedure, which involves less radiation than five traditional X-rays, takes an hour or more.

Magnetic Resonance Imaging (MRI)

This process, introduced in 1980, can produce extremely clear images of the back, not with radiation, but with magnetic and radio waves. The patient is placed on a narrow bed and slid head-first into the tunnel-like—and very noisy—scanner. A magnetic field affects charged particles in the hydrogen atoms of the body's cells, and the particles react to the radio waves, which are analyzed by computer to produce an image. MRIs can "see through" bone and reveal fluid-filled soft tissue in detail. That's why MRIs are favored to confirm diagnoses of suspected soft-tissue (such as nerve) maladies, while CT scans are favored for those of the bones. MRI images can be either cross-sectional or lateral (lengthwise) views.

Because a powerful magnetic field is involved, MRI cannot be used on patients with pacemakers or other metal implants, or on those with intrauterine devices (IUDs).

Open MRI

Although MRI is not an invasive procedure and does not involve any physical pain, lying motionless inside a noisy electromagnetic tube for thirty minutes to two hours can be stressful, especially for those with a claustrophobic bent. Studies published by *The Lancet* and the *Journal of the American Medical Association* report that a third or more of patients experience anxiety because of an MRI; according to *The Lancet,* for one in ten the anxiety reaches a level severe enough to postpone or cancel the test. Earplugs and music have been offered to patients to counter the continuous noise, antianxiety drugs have been tried, and so have experimental movie-viewers and prism glasses to see outside the close confines of the machine.

Open MRI, a more patient-friendly approach to the test, reduces the noise and eliminates the claustrophobia-inspiring conditions associated with conventional, tunnel-like scanners. With open ends and sides, earlier models used lower-strength magnets (one-twelfth as powerful as the standard MRI) that resulted in lower quality images and less detail. The newer open MRIs offer increasingly better magnetic power, and some claim to produce image detail equivalent to the traditional machines.

Less Common Diagnostic Tests

For those whose back pain cannot be explained by any of the more common forms of examination, a variety of other diagnostic tools may be used.

Blood and Urine Tests

Infections, tumors, and diseases—even forms of cancer and arthritis—may be a cause or complication of back pain and can be detected through a variety of blood tests. White and red blood cell

F.Y.I.

Before undergoing diagnostic tests, you can often take the first step in figuring out which category of problem is causing your back pain by paying attention to what kind of movement brings on (or increases) your pain.

• **Strains and sprains.** If you have a strain or sprain, positions that demand extreme ranges of motion, particularly rotation, will increase your pain. So will any kind of jarring move. Strains and sprains usually begin to hurt fairly soon after the injury that caused them.

• **Disk problems.** With a disk problem, flexion and rotation toward one side usually cause the most pain. Occasionally, however, a disk may bulge or herniate centrally, so the pain isn't always one-sided.

(Continued on page 43)

counts, levels of minerals and enzymes all tell a story. If a rheumatoid factor appears, the patient will undergo other tests for rheumatoid arthritis. When a clinical exam leads your doctor to think that the kidneys could be to blame for your back pain, he or she will order urinalysis, which can diagnose infections and other malfunctions of the kidneys.

Bone Scans

Infrequently used in connection with back pain, a bone scan might be taken to detect or rule out bone tumors, differentiate fractures from hidden bone injury, and monitor degenerative bone disorders. A radioactive isotope, or "tracer," is injected into a vein, usually in the arm, and the patient must then be patient—waiting one to three hours while the isotope is absorbed by bone cells and, in that time, drinking several glasses of water or tea. The scan, which takes about an hour, is itself painless, although the positions in which you might have to stay still while you're being scanned might be a bit uncomfortable. The scanner detects rays from the radioactive chemical (which emits less radiation than a standard X-ray machine), and converts them into images that look like X-rays. If a tumor is found, a biopsy will be done to see whether it is malignant or benign. Most tumors are benign.

Diskograms and Diagnostic Blocks

The diskogram is a procedure during which radiopaque dye is injected into a disk suspected of being herniated. X-rays are then taken of the structure of the disk, and the patient's pain response is monitored. If the disk is ruptured, the dye can be seen to escape through the rupture, and will likely reach the nerve root and reproduce the pain.

The diagnostic block is a procedure during which, along with the dye, a numbing anesthetic medication is injected in or around a suspected structure (be it a disk, nerve root, facet joint, or other) in an effort to see whether the pain lessens when the structure is reached.

Electromyography (EMG) and Nerve Conduction Studies

Used both to diagnose neuromuscular disorders and in biofeedback training, an electromyograph converts a muscle's electrical activity into either a visual image or into sound, and measures it to see if the activity—and, thus, the muscle's functional ability—are at normal levels. (The electrocardiogram is an EMG of the heart.)

The test takes about an hour. A metal plate is placed under the patient or near the part of the body being studied, an extremely fine needle electrode is inserted into the muscle in question, and the muscle's electrical activity is measured both at rest and when contracted by the patient. The measurement is amplified one million times and displayed on a screen, and photographs of the image, called electromyograms, are taken. While the sound of a healthy muscle might go from a "putt-putt" to a roar when contracted, a disabled muscle might go from a "putt-putt" to a crackle. Surface electromyography (SEMG) works on the same premise, but uses electrodes placed on the skin instead of needles.

This same machine is used for nerve conduction studies, during which a very low voltage electrical shock is applied through the needle

F.Y.I.

• **Spinal stenosis.** Prolonged extension aggravates spinal stenosis. Pain associated with this problem tends to be chronic.

• **Facet joint problems.** Prolonged extension also tends to increase facet joint problems, which also tend to cause chronic pain. People who experience an acute flare-up in a facet joint usually find rotation increases their pain dramatically.

• **Osteoarthritis.** This kind of pain, like that from strains and sprains, is generally increased by extreme ranges of motion. It will also increase, however, from vibration and compression—for example, jumping up and down. Osteoarthritis pain also tends to develop more slowly; in some cases not until the next day.

Source: The Ultimate Back Book, by Judylaine Fine, Stoddart Publishing Co., Limited, 1997.

electrodes, and the length of time between the stimulation of the nerve and its reaction are measured.

Thermography

Thermography is a noninvasive test that takes about thirty to forty-five minutes and searches for a possible cause of back pain, such as soft-tissue injury or herniated disks, in heat patterns generated by the tissues. The areas to be studied are cooled with room-temperature water, then dried with cool air, and the patient is left to relax for ten to fifteen minutes. An electronic or liquid-crystal thermography apparatus is used to take the thermograms. For lumbar spine studies, thermograms are made of the lower back, buttocks and legs; thoracic or dorsal studies call for thermograms of the mid-back region; and, for cervical spine studies, thermograms would be taken of the back of the neck, the back of the shoulders, and the arms.

Cerebrospinal Fluid (CSF) Analysis

Also known as a spinal tap, this test is used to confirm diagnosis of central nervous system infections, hemorrhage, or tumors that might be blocking the circulation of cerebrospinal fluid, which helps maintain pressure within the spinal cord and brain. The patient lies on her side on a table, with knees pulled up toward the chin. A local anesthetic is injected, and then a needle is inserted into the spinal canal to collect the fluid. Pressure of the fluid is measured before and after collection, and the fluid is sent to a lab for analysis. After the test, the patient remains lying flat on the back for a lengthy period of time, without raising the head. The test usually takes less than an hour, and a headache is the most common side effect.

Spinal Endoscopy

Also called epiduroscopy or epidural spinal endoscopy, this relatively new technique for examining soft tissue (approved by the Food and Drug Administration as a diagnostic tool in 1996) uses fiberoptic and video technology to allow physicians to physically and visually explore the interior of the spine without surgery.

During the hour-long procedure, performed while the patient is sedated but awake, a small incision is made at the base of the tailbone. After the area is numbed, a flexible fiberoptic endoscope the diameter of a toothpick is threaded into the space between the spinal cord and the vertebrae via a steerable catheter, a tube about the width of a ballpoint pen refill. Not only can the doctor view the spinal interior in full color on a video monitor, allowing certain conditions (such as red inflamed nerve roots, for instance) to be more readily identified, but he can physically move tissue in search of the problem and receive feedback from the patient as to whether he's reached the source of the pain. Since receiving additional FDA approval as a delivery system for medication in 1998, spinal endoscopy can also be used to treat some of the problems it detects.

Although it is not as invasive as surgery, endoscopy is more invasive than other diagnostic tests and is used for the most part only when surgery is the only alternative and when your doctor believes you can benefit from the administration of medication while he's "inside."

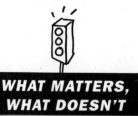

WHAT MATTERS, WHAT DOESN'T

What Matters
• Knowing which signs and symptoms call for a visit to the doctor.

• Finding an experienced health care practitioner you can trust.

• Recognizing that abnormal test results don't necessarily identify the cause of your pain.

What Doesn't
• Knowing the specific bodily structures involved in causing the pain.

• Limiting your care to only one specialist.

• High-tech diagnostic tests performed prematurely.

Before taking any diagnostic test, be sure to follow your doctor's instructions about pretest food restrictions or fasting, the intake of fluids and/or caffeine, smoking, activity levels, and any other advisories that can affect test results and your safety. Tell your doctor whether you're pregnant, of course, and whether you have any allergies—even to iodine or shellfish if your test involves the injection of any dyes.

Although you may never know the specific cause of much of your own back pains, a familiarity with some of the more common problems, and when they are likely to appear, can help. The next chapter takes a look at how.

THE BOTTOM LINE

As elusive to find the source of as it is common to occur, back pain is not an easily diagnosable ill. The good news is that we don't necessarily need to know exactly where it's coming from in order to find relief. What we do need to know are the warning signs and symptoms of a serious problem, and what our doctors can—and cannot—do to help.

What Can Go Wrong— and When

Back pain can be blamed on everything from injuries to disease. Some of the causes stem from being out of shape, some from moving incorrectly, and some from what happens to our bodies as we age. Back pain may be caused by a sprain or strain; or it may be caused by hours spent inert on the couch, which is why muscles often are so easily "strainable" to begin with.

In this chapter we start out by taking a look at just some of the many things that can go wrong— not for the purpose of scaring ourselves into a hypochondriacal frenzy, but to get an idea of what can go wrong and when, what can be prevented and how, and what can be eased and what can be healed.

What Can Go Wrong

Back pain can be divided into two main types: the first, mechanical back pain (also known as *musculoskeletal back pain*) involves strains, sprains, and any other injury that doesn't cause damage to the nerves. Compressive pain (also called *neurogenic pain*) occurs when the nerve roots of the spine are irritated or pinched. Among the symptoms that the nerves are involved are pain and numbness or weakness in the area supplied by the nerve, which can extend into the arms, or down below the knee. Traditionally, orthopedic surgeons treated mechanical back pain, and neurosurgeons handled compressive problems, but increasingly, the lines are blurred.

The people who experience back pain can be divided into three main types. Loren M. Fishman,

M.D., of Columbia University College of Physicians and Surgeons and Albert Einstein College of Medicine in New York, categorizes them as, "People with normal backs doing abnormal activity, people with abnormal backs doing normal activity, or people doing normal activity for which they're not prepared."

Although back pain might seem to come "out of the blue," chances are it's been easing its way over the horizon for quite some time. Cumulative stress on bones and soft tissue adds up, and wears us down—degeneration occurs. You might *think* it was that heavy suitcase that put your back "out," but the overall condition of the spine and its support structure—which your lifestyle has been affecting, one way or the other, for years—are the real cause. And the condition of that spine and support structure is what's going to determine how fast you will recover, too.

As for exactly what's to blame, we might never know. "For about 85 percent of people we don't have a clearly identifiable cause of the pain," says David M. Montgomery, M.D., an orthopedic surgeon specializing in the spine at William Beaumont Hospital in Royal Oak, Michigan. "We have a general idea, but can't find anything definitive."

"The exact cause often eludes us," seconds Richard S. Materson, M.D., professor of physical medicine and rehabilitation at Baylor College of Medicine and University of Texas Health Science Center. "There are lots and lots of things that can happen that make it seem like the back is mad at us."

Following are some of the main causes. We tried to put them into tidy categories, but there is considerable overlap. Someone with spinal stenosis, a narrowing of the spinal canal, is more susceptible to pain from a herniated disk or bone

SMART DEFINITION

Strain

Stretched or torn muscle or tendon.

Sprain

The violent overstretching or tearing of one or more ligaments.

spur. Alternatively, the troublesome disks or bone spurs might be responsible for the narrowing of the spinal canal. Inflammation or muscle spasm might compound the effect. Keep in mind, too, that many of these conditions can be found in people with no back pain at all. Just because you have a bulging disk doesn't mean you'll be in pain.

We start with the most common causes of back pain—strains and sprains—and list the remainder in alphabetical order.

Strains and Sprains

The most common causes of low back pain by far, strains and sprains can be confusing. Even different types of doctors and medical dictionaries disagree. According to the *Merriam-Webster Medical Dictionary* and some physicians, strain involves an overstretching of muscles, tendons, or ligaments, while sprain involves a tearing of those tissues.

But ask an orthopedic surgeon, and you'll learn that a strain is a stretched or torn muscle or tendon, the cord or band of fibrous connective tissue that attaches the muscle to the bone; while a sprain is the violent overstretching or tearing of one or more ligaments, the tissue that attaches bone to bone.

Strains tend to occur when muscles are poorly conditioned and/or overworked. If, for example, you're out of shape and spend an entire weekend raking leaves in the garden, stretching to get into hard-to-reach places, twisting to load the trash bags, and the next day you feel as if you cannot move a muscle, chances are you have a strain. Chronic strains are caused by overuse (too many hours of work in a row). Acute strains are caused by direct injury or overstress (picking up something that's too heavy).

Sprains tend to happen when a sudden, forceful movement (a sudden or violent twist or wrench) injures a ligament, which is more susceptible if it's stiff or weak through poor conditioning or overuse. Ligaments are not as flexible as muscles and tendons, and are more susceptible to tearing. When the ligament is overstretched, it becomes tense and gives way at its weakest point, either where it attaches to bone or within the ligament itself. Sprains usually occur because of trauma—a fall, a twisting injury, or an accident—that ruptures blood vessels at the same time. They are recognizable by severe pain at the time of the injury, swelling, inflammation, and discoloration.

Both strains and sprains are categorized into three types, from Grade I (mild) to Grade III (severe). Mild strains (Grade I) involve a slightly pulled muscle without tearing of muscle or tendon fibers, and no loss of strength; moderate strains (Grade II) tear fibers in a muscle, tendon, or at the attachment to bone, and cause diminished strength; and severe (Grade III) strains rupture the muscle-tendon-bone attachment with separation of fibers.

Mild (Grade I) sprains involve the tearing of some ligament fibers, but no loss of function; moderate (Grade II) sprains rupture part of the ligament, causing some functional loss; and severe (Grade III) sprains cause complete rupture of the ligament or complete separation of ligament from bone.

If you're still uncertain about which is which, you're not alone. Even diagnostically, it can be difficult to differentiate the two. Both may cause pain or tenderness; with sprains and the more severe strains causing swelling; and redness or bruising either immediately or several hours later. "If the pain gets worse on the second or third day, and then starts to improve, [a strain or a sprain] might be the cause," says Dr. Fishman. Other clues that it's a strain or a sprain: pressing the area hurts, pain is activated by a specific movement, or a massage or warm bath makes it feel better.

Here are some helpful hints for preventing and treating strains and sprains:

• **Lower your risk.** Don't overtax yourself with more physical activity than your body is ready for. Maintain a good level of physical fitness and proper weight, and stretch muscles before and after exercise.

• **If necessary, use over-the-counter pain relievers.** Acetaminophen or ibuprofen can help reduce the pain.

• **Treat yourself right.** Follow the dos and don'ts for acute and chronic back pain in chapter 2.

• **Avoid repeat performances.** You might not be able to figure out exactly which tendon or ligament is hurting, but narrowing down the cause to the new workout routine, office chair, or even that new pair of high heels can prevent recurrence. "About 80 percent of back pain is musculoskeletal, which means it will probably go away on its own," says Dr. Fishman. "But whatever you did to make it happen—do it again and it will happen again."

Arachnoiditis

Arachnoiditis is one of the less common causes of back pain, though without question a serious disease. An inflammation of the arachnoid—an extremely thin, spider-web-like membrane sandwiched between two other membranes, or meninges, that cover and protect the brain and spinal cord—arachnoiditis can result from infection (for example, meningitis, tuberculosis, or syphilis); or trauma, including trauma resulting from surgery, lumbar puncture, or spinal anesthesia. Besides surgery, the most common cause is the introduction of chemicals into the spinal canal, and the most severe effects have been linked with an oil-based dye formerly used for myelograms. (Such dyes, used as recently as 1991, have been replaced with safer, water-soluble dyes today.)

Sometimes diagnosed as "failed back syndrome," arachnoiditis can appear soon or many years after the incident that prompted it, causing the membranes encasing the spinal cord to become thickened and scarred, and then trapping the nerve roots within the scar tissue. Cysts and other complications may occur. The pain is frequently described as a burning or stinging sensation in the back and down one or more limbs as far as the ankles and feet, and it often persists during rest. Depending on the severity of the disease, symptoms can include headaches, seizures, blindness, or progressive paralysis. There may be bladder, bowel, and sexual dysfunction; muscle spasms; rashes; itching; and numbness.

There is no cure for this often disabling disease, and some symptoms may become permanent. Conservative therapy such as pain management is generally recommended, because even in patients

SMART DEFINITION

Arachnoiditis

Inflammation of one of the membranes that encase and protect the brain and spinal cord.

whose disease is worsening, surgery to remove scar tissue won't stop new scar tissue from developing. Also, surgery exposes the already irritated spinal cord to additional trauma.

Facet Joint Problems

Less common than disk problems (and they are not as common as we tend to think), problems of the facet joints—the joints between the vertebrae—can be caused or exacerbated by the changes that occur in aging disks.

In chapter 1 we described facets as being the smooth faces on the ends of the articular processes, the bony parts of each vertebra that help "connect" it to the vertebrae above and below. The processes join at the facet joint, which is encased in a joint capsule that keeps the facets together, but allows them to move. Cartilage capping the facets allows them to move smoothly.

As the disks dry out and flatten with age, allowing the vertebrae to settle closer together, the facets come closer as well. The result: when the facet joints settle, they can end up rubbing against each other when they move, and the cartilage becomes worn, allowing irritation, impeding function, and causing pain. Weakened or stretched muscle tissue can also take its toll. If muscles can't adequately support the facet joints, the joints end up bearing more weight, and the same kind of settling occurs. Facet joint syndrome can result.

One symptom of facet joint problems is pain when you extend your back (arch backward), which brings the joints closer together. Dull, "nonspecific" leg pain is another symptom.

Other facet joint problems can be prompted by

sudden twists of the body, causing the joint capsule to get caught and bruised by the joint. Inflammation and muscle spasm can result. In addition, rapidly dropping barometric pressure before a storm is thought by some to cause fluid in the capsule to expand, causing pain.

Fibromyalgia

SMART DEFINITION

Fibromyalgia

A rheumatologic disorder that affects the muscles and soft tissues.

Like rheumatoid arthritis and osteoporosis (see below), fibromyalgia is a rheumatologic disorder, which means it is characterized by inflammation and pain in muscles and joints. But while osteoarthritis and rheumatoid arthritis affect joints, fibromyalgia affects the muscles and soft tissues. Symptoms are wide-ranging, from muscle ache and stiffness, fatigue, and headaches to disturbed sleep, depression, and tingling in the extremities; and it has been estimated to affect up to 5 percent of the population.

The American College of Rheumatology's diagnostic guideline to tell whether a person has fibromyalgia specifies both widespread general pain (defined as pain on both sides of the body, above and below the waist, and spinal pain) for at least three months; and pain in eleven of eighteen tender point sites. "For a tender point to be considered 'positive,'" read the guidelines, "the subject must state that the palpation was painful. 'Tender' is not to be considered 'painful.'"

Because there are no specific lab tests to accurately diagnose it, however, fibromyalgia has been the source of some controversy, with many scientists and physicians speculating it is not a physical disorder because no telltale abnormalities could be found in tissues or blood. Recent research at the University of Alabama at Birmingham, however, found people with fibromyalgia have a diminished flow of blood to parts of the brain, and an increase in a chemical substance that helps transmit pain signals.

"This finding should provide some relief to millions of people who've been told that their pain is all in their head," said Laurence Bradley, Ph.D., who led the study.

If you suspect you have fibromyalgia, you'll probably be referred to a rheumatologist, who is a medical specialist trained in the field of rheumatologic disease. Treatment therapies have involved antidepressants and gentle exercise, stress management, and a diet rich in carbohydrates.

Fractures and Breaks

Fractures or breaks of the bones of the spine can occur due to a variety of sources, not the least of which is trauma inflicted by accidents and physical injury. Fortunately, the muscles of the back protect the spine well, so we're much less likely to break a vertebra than, say, our arm with a simple fall. Disease, on the other hand, renders us more susceptible: osteoporosis alone is responsible for more than 700,000 vertebral fractures every year.

• **Stress fractures.** Also known as *fatigue fractures,* these hairline breaks in the bone can be caused by direct or indirect stress on the bone and tend to develop over long periods of time. Although they do not require setting, they can cause pressure on or injury to nearby nerves, joints, ligaments, and tendons, and staying active after symptoms start puts you at risk for more severe fracture and damage. Contact sports increase the risk, as does a history of bone or joint disease (especially osteoporosis), obesity, and a calcium-deficient diet. Signs and symptoms include pain in the injured area, swelling and bruising of soft tissue around it, tenderness, the feeling of warmth over the site, and sometimes numbness beyond the fracture site. Average healing time is six to eight weeks.

• **Spondylolysis and spondylolisthesis.** Both of these conditions involve a crack in the vertebra, and, surprisingly enough, both can exist without our knowing they are there. *Spondylolysis,* a hairline fracture across the back of the vertebra, is almost undetectable, and it's been estimated that as many as 20 percent of us have a mild case. We can be born with a tendency to develop spondylolysis, and prolonged stress on the bone can make it happen. But it usually doesn't cause pain or trouble until it progresses to the much more infrequent *spondylolisthesis,* where the hairline crack widens. And if it widens enough, the front part of the vertebra detaches from the rear and can gradually begin to slip forward. Even severe cases can respond to non-surgical treatment, although surgery is an option in extremes.

Herniated and Bulging Disks

The intervertebral disks that serve so well as spinal column shock absorbers most of our lives can be the cause of trouble as we—and they—age. This problem goes by many names: ruptured, prolapsed, or protruding disk; the scientific-sounding herniated nucleus pulposus; and the erroneous but oft-used "slipped disk" (the spinal structure

SMART DEFINITION

Herniated or ruptured disk

A disk in which the outer shell has torn due to degeneration or trauma, allowing the soft inner core to protrude into the spinal canal.

Bulging disk

A disk in which the inner core intrudes into a rupture within the outer shell, but does not extend beyond the surface of the disk.

Slipped disk

A commonly used but anatomically incorrect term referring to herniated disks.

holds the disks firmly in place; they do not "slip" anywhere).

"During life, the disk goes from being a very fluid-filled, movable shock absorber to basically a piece of bone that doesn't have movement or shock absorption abilities," says Dr. Richard Materson. Basically, two things happen. The soft inner core (nucleus pulposus), which had a jellylike consistency during youth, begins to take on the fibrous nature of the disk's tough outer shell (annulus fibrosus). Meanwhile, through wear and trauma, the outer tissue can tear, allowing material from the disk to push out, or rupture, into the spinal canal. Sometimes, the material doesn't fully escape, but merely causes the disk to bulge.

It may come as a surprise to learn that none of this necessarily causes any pain at all. The pain happens not from the herniation or bulge itself, but when the herniation or bulge causes the disk to press on a nerve root, irritating or pinching it. The pain is not always felt in the back; it is common to experience the problem along the path of the nerve. A herniated lumbar disk, for example, typically produces sciatica—pain down the back of the leg, sometimes extending to the side of the calf, and sometimes into the side of the foot. Sensory and/or motor function of the affected nerve root can also be impaired, causing numbness or weakness in the areas served by the nerve.

Disks of the neck or lower spine are the most common sites for ruptured or protruding disks. Lumbar disk problems almost always involve the three lowest disks—95 percent of the time, the lower two—and in the vast majority of cases, the nerve root being compressed is the one exiting the level below.

Pain tends to be sharp and specific and worsens with movement. If the problem is in the lumbar spine, you'd feel severe pain in the low back or the back of one leg, the buttock, or even the calf down to the foot. Pain usually affects one side, and coughing, sneezing, lifting, or straining can make it worse. You might also feel weakness in or numbness of the leg. If a cervical disk in the neck is involved, you'd feel pain in the neck, shoulder, or down one arm, with possible weakness or numbness in that arm.

"Disk ruptures usually heal without surgery, but slowly," says Dr. David Montgomery, who notes that many patients opt for surgery nevertheless. "It's often a quality of life issue. People can't stand pain and disability for a year or two, but want surgery to get better quickly and move on with life."

Inflammation

Like muscle spasms, inflammation is one of the body's ways of taking care of itself, and you will see it listed as a result and/or symptom of many of the maladies listed here. This automatic response to infection from invading bacteria or viruses, disease, or injury is a healing process marked by enlargement of the tiny blood vessels (capillaries) in the affected area, redness, heat, swelling, pain, and sometimes loss of function, that helps the body eliminate poisons and heal damaged tissue.

Muscle Spasm

Caused by anything from emotional stress to the body's effort to protect a damaged part by keeping it immobilized, muscle spasms are involuntary,

SMART DEFINITION

Inflammation

Enlargement of tiny blood vessels known as capillaries, marked by redness, swelling, heat, and/or pain.

Muscle spasm

An involuntary, sustained and sometimes immobilizing contraction of the elastic tissues that support the bones and allow the body to move.

SMART DEFINITION

Myofascial pain syndrome (MPS)

A chronic, generalized ache of the muscles and connective tissues that doesn't have a detectable cause.

Osteoarthritis

A breakdown of the cushioning of the joints often associated with the wear-and-tear of aging.

powerful, and sustained contractions of muscle or muscle fibers. They are a very common cause of pain, and are associated with many of the problems described in this chapter.

Normal muscle contractions are what allow us to move and occur when nerve fibers relay messages from the brain to the muscles to tell them to contract—or shorten. Muscle spasms happen when the muscles contract too much, for too long, and not from conscious effort. The pain comes, in part, from the direct effect of muscle spasm on mechanically sensitive pain receptors. The muscle "squeezes" the pain receptors, like someone squeezing your arm, and that hurts. Muscle spasm can also cause pain indirectly by compressing blood vessels, which decreases blood flow and denies oxygen to tissues, which in turn stimulates chemically sensitive pain receptors. The muscle spasm also increases the rate of metabolism (the energy-burning capacity) in the muscle tissue at the same time, which makes the tissue need more oxygen at the same time as it is being deprived of it. *Ouch.*

Myofascial Pain Syndrome (MPS)

In several ways resembling fibromyalgia, with which it is often associated, myofascial pain syndrome is characterized by a chronic, generalized ache that occurs in the muscles and connective tissues without a detectable cause and provokes tenderness at soft tissue sites. Unlike fibromyalgia's "tender points," however, MPS *trigger points* cause referred pain—you hurt in an area other than the trigger point site, and not necessarily along the path of the nerve associated with the area. Another diagnostic signal is the local *twitch response:* an involuntary muscle movement that sometimes occurs when a finger is rolled over the trigger point.

Treatment for myofascial pain is mostly non-medicinal, with physical therapy, muscle stretching, and massage playing the major roles.

Osteoarthritis

Dubbed "the wear-and-tear arthritis," osteoarthritis (OA) causes the breakdown of the joint's cartilage, which is the part of the joint that cushions the ends of bones. Cartilage breakdown causes bones to rub against each other, causing pain and loss of movement. One of the most common types of arthritis, affecting one in seven Americans (mostly after age forty-five and more often women than men), OA is also called degenerative arthritis, degenerative joint disease, or hypertrophic arthritis, and it particularly affects hands and weight-bearing joints such as those found in the back, knees, hips, and feet.

Although the exact cause is not known, genetics play a role in who is more susceptible to early cartilage breakdown. Other risk factors include obesity, previous joint injuries, and jobs that put stress on joints. Although age is a risk factor, doctors now know that OA is a disease, rather than part of "natural aging." Most people over sixty reveal the disease on X-ray, but only about one-third of those with positive X-rays have actual symptoms.

Effects range from very mild to severe joint stiffness and pain and can include limited movement and loss of dexterity, sometimes swelling of

SMART SOURCES

Arthritis Foundation
1330 West Peachtree St.
Atlanta, GA 30309
800-283-7800
404-872-7100
www.arthritis.org

This is the only national, voluntary health organization dedicated to the nearly 43 million people who have any of the more than one hundred forms of arthritis or related diseases. Nationwide chapters offer self-help courses, exercise classes, support groups, videotapes and free brochures, and the bimonthly consumer magazine *Arthritis Today.*

SMART DEFINITION

Osteophyte

A buildup of excess bone, also referred to as a bone spur.

Osteoporosis

A decrease in bone density and strength, and a common cause of fracture, especially among postmenopausal women.

affected joints, and cracking or grating sounds with joint movement. Weather changes, especially to cold, damp weather, may increase the ache.

Treatment focuses on decreasing pain and improving joint movement. Acetaminophen can help reduce mild pain without inflammation; and non-steroidal anti-inflammatory drugs (NSAIDs), including aspirin, are recommended if there is inflammation or the acetaminophen doesn't help. Other treatments include use of heat or cold for temporary pain relief; exercises to keep joints flexible; and weight control to prevent extra stress on joints. Recently, the National Institutes of Health concluded that acupuncture can be an alternative or addition to conventional osteoarthritis care. In severe cases, surgery is another option.

Osteoarthritis should not be confused with *rheumatoid arthritis* (RA), a disease of the autoimmune system that attacks many joints throughout the body simultaneously and often begins between the ages of twenty-five and fifty but can occur in children as early as infancy. Developing within weeks or months, rheumatoid arthritis usually affects small joints of the hands and feet, causing redness, warmth and swelling. Symptoms can include general feelings of sickness and fatigue, as well as weight loss and fever; and prolonged morning stiffness. An antibody called a *rheumatoid factor* may be found in the blood. For this, and all types of arthritis, a rheumatologist is the medical professional to see.

Osteophytes

Osteophytes, also referred to as bone spurs, a build-up of bone on the vertebrae, are blamed for pinched nerves and for the narrowing of the spinal canal called spinal stenosis, among other things. Very common, and increasing in number and size with age, they are just as likely to appear in the pain-free back as in the back that aches.

Osteoporosis

The rheumatologic disorder of osteoporosis, or "porous bone," is the major cause of bone fractures in the elderly, especially postmenopausal women. Marked by a decrease in bone mass and strength, its most predictable medical cause in women is menopause, when estrogen levels drop, but a variety of factors can cause the appearance of osteoporosis at a younger age. According to the National Osteoporosis Foundation, the disease "is a major public health threat for more than 28 million Americans, 80 percent of whom are women."

One in two women and one in eight men over age fifty will have an osteoporosis-related fracture in their lifetime, and the disease is responsible for more than 1.5 million fractures annually, including approximately 700,000 of the vertebrae.

The best treatment for osteoporosis is prevention. The more bone mass you have, the more strength you have, and the lower the risk of fracture. And it's never too late to "bone up." A three-year study of men and women over age sixty-five found that those who took calcium and vitamin D

SMART SOURCES

National Osteoporosis Foundation
1150 17th Street NW, Suite 500
Washington, D.C. 20036
202-223-2226
www.nof.org

This resource provides up-to-date information on the causes, prevention, detection and treatment of osteoporosis. Members receive a quarterly newsletter and a copy of the handbook, *Boning Up on Osteoporosis*. A variety of brochures and educational materials are available to the public for a small fee.

SMART DEFINITION

Pinched nerves

A nerve that is compressed by another anatomical structure, such as a disk or osteophyte.

Sacroiliac joint problems

Pain related to the straining of ligaments connecting the sacrum (the spinal bone below the moveable vertebrae) and the ilia (the hip bones).

supplements daily had less than half as many broken bones as the placebo group.

To ward off the effects of osteoporosis, we're advised to eat a healthy diet that fulfills requirements of calcium and vitamins and limits or eliminates alcohol, caffeine, and tobacco (read more about nutrition on page 83). It also helps to take part in lower-extremity exercises such as walking and back extension exercises to stabilize or slightly increase bone mass, improve balance, and strengthen muscles. Estrogen replacement therapies have also been found helpful in preventing postmenopausal bone loss.

Pinched Nerves

Compressive or neurogenic pain caused by a "pinched" or compressed nerve can occur as the result of many factors—the narrowing of the spinal canal called spinal stenosis, herniated disks, or osteophytes, many of which are described in their own sections here. If the compression lasts long enough, the result can be the *absence* of pain when the doctor tests for it (called objective numbness).

Sacroiliac Joint Problems

On each side of the sacrum, the arrowhead-shaped bone between the moveable vertebrae and the coccyx, are ligaments attaching it to the ilia, the two large bones of the pelvis, or hip bones. And what joins them are the sacroiliac joints. Straining of those ligaments can cause a very specific, localized pain that usually becomes worse when sitting and is usually relieved by walking. It is very common during pregnancy, when hormones allow more movement in the joints than normally occurs (see page 81). Physical manipulation of the joints by a health care professional will often provide relief.

Scoliosis

In addition to the natural forward and backward curves of the spine, people with scoliosis have spines that curve side to side, resembling an "S" or "C" when viewed straight on, rather than a straight line. Some of the bones also may have rotated slightly, making the waist or shoulders appear uneven.

Eighty-five percent of cases are idiopathic, meaning "no known cause," and usually appear in early adolescent boys and girls, although girls are five to eight times more likely to have the curves increase in size and require treatment. Heredity might play a role in the disease, but exactly what role is yet to be known. Several other, less common, types of scoliosis have known causes, including birth defects, central nervous system and muscle diseases (such as muscular dystrophy), and disorders of connective tissue (Marfan's syndrome).

In 90 percent of cases, the curvature is mild enough not to require active treatment; and most treatment to date is helpful only to still-developing spines. Adolescents should be monitored for change, and evaluation by an orthopedic surgeon will determine if an orthopedic back brace is required—not to make the spine straight, but to stop the curves from getting worse. In a small number of patients, surgery is undertaken to improve the deformity and prevent it from progressing.

SMART SOURCES

Spina Bifida Association
 of America
4590 MacArthur Blvd.
 N.W., No. 250
Washington, D.C.
 20007
800-621-3141
202-944-3285
www.sbaa.org

Spina Bifida and Hydro-
 cephalus Association
 of Canada
220–388 Donald St.
Winnipeg, Manitoba
Canada R3B 2J4
800-565-9488
204-925-3650
www.sbhac.ca

These nonprofit organi-
zations offer a wealth
of information and
support to people with
spina bifida, their
family members, and
the general public.

Scoliosis is not usually painful in adolescence, but can become so in adulthood. For minor discomfort from muscle imbalance or complications, nonprescription drugs such as aspirin or acetaminophen are recommended. Physical exercises and activities may be part of therapy to tone and strengthen the back and improve posture.

Spina Bifida

The most common birth defect, affecting one of every one thousand infants born in the United States and one of every 750 newborns in Canada, spina bifida is a neural tube defect (NTD) in which the back of the spinal column does not completely close during fetal development, causing varying degrees of damage to the spinal cord and nervous system.

In its most severe form, *myelomeningocele,* the spinal cord protrudes from the opening in the spine. In its mildest form, *spina bifida occulta* (meaning "hidden"), the defect might involve only one or more malformed vertebrae, with an opening so miniscule it can barely be detected. Depending upon the degree of severity, spina bifida can cause almost no problem, or extensive disability, including bowel and bladder disorders, walking dysfunction or paralysis, and learning disabilities. A large percentage of children born with spina bifida also have *hydrocephalus,* an accumulation of fluid in the brain.

Although there is no single known cause, adequate intake of folic acid, a B vitamin, prior to and during the first trimester of pregnancy can significantly reduce the risk of this and other neural tube defects—cutting their incidence by as much as 75 percent. Because it occurs in the first four weeks of pregnancy, before a woman might even know she is pregnant, all women capable of becoming pregnant are advised to consume 0.4 milligrams of folic acid daily, the amount in most daily multivitamin supplements. Those with a previous NTD-affected pregnancy or a close family history of NTDs should consult their physician about increasing that amount.

Treatment for the more severe forms of spina bifida includes surgery, medication, physiotherapy, and the use of assistive devices.

Spinal Stenosis

The word *stenosis* refers to the narrowing or constriction of the diameter of a bodily passage. Spinal stenosis is the narrowing of the spinal canal, the passage in which the nerves are located. It usually occurs in either the lumbar or cervical (low back or neck) areas due to either a problem you're born with, or one that develops in older age. The condition can cause pain when the narrowing results in a nerve being irritated or pinched by surrounding parts of the spine.

A small percentage of us are born with unusually narrow spinal canals (less than half an inch wide), allowing less room through which the nerves can freely pass. For others, the narrowing occurs in middle or older age from a variety of causes, including the development of bony formations (osteophytes or bone spurs) along the vertebrae; and the normal degeneration of the disks, which causes vertebrae and soft tissue to move inward toward the spinal canal. As you might imagine, those who start out with an already narrow

SMART DEFINITION

Spina bifida

A birth defect in which the back of the spinal column doesn't completely close during prenatal development.

Spinal stenosis

A narrowing of the spinal canal, usually occurring in either the low back or neck area.

SMART SOURCES

Spondylitis Association
of America
14827 Ventura Blvd.,
Suite 222
Sherman Oaks, CA
91403
800-777-8189
www.spondylitis.org

The largest resource for
information on anky-
losing spondylitis and
related diseases in the
United States, SAA
offers support, network-
ing opportunities, and
rheumatologist referral.
Self-help information is
offered in the form of a
newsletter, pamphlets,
books, videos and
audiotapes. A free
information package is
available by calling the
toll-free information
line.

space are at a disadvantage. Injury to the spine or a malformed vertebra can also be to blame.

If the trouble is in the lumbar spine, symptoms can include pain in the buttocks, thigh, and calf; progressive numbness or weakness in the leg, which, like the pain, might worsen with activity; and bladder and bowel problems. If the problem is in the cervical spine, symptoms are likely to appear in the shoulders and arms.

Different types of spinal stenosis—central, segmental, lateral, and others—refer to different areas and causes of narrowing.

Spondylitis

Spondylitis refers to any inflammation of the spine. In many cases it can be caused by infection, either elsewhere in the body, or from an infected incision during back surgery. A reaction to a chemical injected into the spine is another cause. The standard treatment is antibiotics and rest.

Spondylitis is also used as the shorthand term for ankylosing spondylitis (AS) or Marie-Strumpell disease, a rare form of arthritis that primarily involves the spine and joints of the shoulders, hips, and knees. It tends to strike young adults, and twice as many men as women are affected. About one million Americans have the disease, which causes pain, stiffness, and, in very severe cases, a fusing of the vertebrae starting at the base of the spine and progressing upward.

Although the cause of AS is not known, a link has been made to a gene called HLA-B27, with which 8 percent of us are born. Only 2 percent of that small group will eventually get AS, which researchers believe might be triggered by a bacterial infection of the intestines.

Early warning signs of AS, according to the Spondylitis Association of America (SAA), are onset of pain before the age of thirty-five; early morning stiffness of the spine; improvement of discomfort with mild activity or a hot shower; back pain that starts gradually; and duration of symptoms longer than three months. Patients almost always have at least four of these five symptoms, says SAA.

Although there is no cure, treatment with non-steroidal anti-inflammatory drugs (NSAIDs) such as aspirin and other medications, regular exercise, good posture and relaxation habits, and education can help. With proper diagnosis and treatment, the more severe problems can usually be prevented or minimized, and most people continue to lead physically active lives.

Tumors

Although they are fortunately among the less-common causes of back pain, tumors and cancers of the back certainly merit discussion. Whether benign (noncancerous) or malignant (cancerous), a tumor of the spinal cord can compress the spine or nerve roots, wreaking considerable damage unless appropriately and swiftly treated. Benign bone tumors are more common than malignant ones, but both types can grow and damage healthy bone tissue.

There are many kinds of tumors. *Meningiomas*— affecting the membranes that surround the brain and spinal cord—account for about 50 percent of primary brain and spinal cord tumors. About 85 percent are benign and curable by surgery. *Chordo-*

SMART DEFINITION

Spondylitis

Any inflammation of the spine. Ankylosing spondylitis, a rare form of arthritis that primarily involves the spine, is believed to have a genetic cause.

Tumors

One of the less common sources of back pain, an abnormal mass of tissue, or growth, that can be benign (noncancerous) or, less frequently, malignant (cancerous).

F.Y.I.

Traumatic Spinal Cord Injury

Number of new injuries per year in the U.S.:
   7,800–10,000
Total number of people with spinal cord injury or spinal dysfunction:
   250,000–400,000

Gender:
   82 percent male
   18 percent female

Highest per capita rate of injury by age:
   Between 16 and 30

Causes of Spinal Cord Injury

Motor vehicle accidents:
   44 percent
Acts of violence:
   24 percent
Falls:
   22 percent*
Sports:
   8 percent (two-thirds from diving)
Other:
   2 percent

* Falls overtake motor vehicles as the leading cause of injury after age 45.
Source: National Spinal Cord Injury Association

mas are tumors that start in the bone at the back of the skull or at the lower end of the spinal cord. Although they typically return many times, they usually do not spread to other organs. *Lymphomas* start in cells of the immune system. Recent advances in chemotherapy have dramatically improved their prognosis. Thirty-seven-year-old Atlanta Braves first baseman Fernando Galarraga was diagnosed with non-Hodgkin's lymphoma of the lumbar vertebrae after a bout of back pain. His treatment: a course of chemotherapy and radiation lasting several months.

Primary cancers (those that begin at the site itself) are rare in the spinal cord and bone; *secondary* or *metastatic cancers* (resulting from cancer that has spread, or metastasized, from another part of the body) are more common. And that makes a difference in treatment. Cancer that arises in the bone (primary bone cancer), for instance, is not the same disease as cancer that spreads to the bone from another part of the body (secondary or metastatic bone cancer).

Chronic back pain that won't go away with conservative treatment, progressive weakness and numbness, and bowel or bladder problems are some of the signs and symptoms that a tumor might be to blame. Bone scans, blood tests, X-rays, MRIs, and biopsy can help confirm the diagnosis; and chemotherapy, radiation therapy, and surgery—along with physical therapy and rehabilitation—are among the treatment options available today.

Early detection of all cancers is key to treatment success. The American Cancer Society recommends women undergo yearly Pap tests for cervical cancer, and beginning at age forty, annual screening mammograms for breast cancer; annual digital rectal exams for colorectal cancers are recommended for all men age forty and up. Beginning at age fifty, both men and women should have yearly tests for colorectal cancers, and men should have an annual prostate specific antigen blood test. People at different levels of risk have different needs. Consult with your physician for the right schedule of preventive care.

When We're Most Susceptible

Just as not all of us are at the same risk of back pain, not all of us face the same level of susceptibility at all times. Factors from weather conditions to turbulent emotions have an affect, as do sleeping patterns and hectic work seasons. Preparing ourselves for those higher risk situations can reduce their impact and the pain that comes with it—or even prevent an injury or pain from happening altogether.

When We're Under Stress

When you feel as though you are "carrying the world on your shoulders," your body might be responding as though you literally are. Emotional stress can lead to physical tension. Your muscles clench and spasm, your posture changes, and your shoulders tighten to bear that heavy load.

Emotional factors can be found at the root of both chronic and acute aches. Even positive life events or changes can be to blame—back trouble can be prompted by the tension that, say, an upcoming wedding or job change brings along.

F.Y.I.

Know the signs of stress:

• Change in appetite

• Change in sleeping patterns

• Skin outbreaks

• Shortened temper

• Change in sexual appetite

• Forgetfulness or absentmindedness

• Increase in smoking or drinking of alcohol

• Change in weight

• Difficulty breathing

• Recurring colds, illnesses, or chronic infections

• Trembling

• Excessive perspiration

• Heart palpitations

Emotional stress impacts the body in two main ways: by its physical effect on our body, which can cause pain directly or leave us more susceptible to other injuries; and by its effect on our actions, which tend to be less carefully undertaken, and more likely to bring about harm.

Stress can make us sick. There is evidence of its role in gastrointestinal, dermatological, respiratory, and neurologic ills, as well as a wide range of infections and immune system disorders—from the common cold and herpes to arthritis and cancer. Headaches, chest pain, shortness of breath, rashes, high blood pressure, indigestion, and insomnia are just some of the results.

The musculoskeletal system is not exempt. Stress has been linked to muscle aches and weakening, arthritis and bone loss, and even higher levels of fat deposits in the body, especially around the abdomen, taxing the spine.

And if that's not enough, there is no question that stress can harm us via the self-destructive behaviors it can provoke. Smoking, drinking, substance abuse, bad diet, and lack of exercise are direct links to ill health associated with stress. And we are likely to drive faster, and dumber, when stressed, increasing the chances of having an accident.

Stress can make pain feel worse and last longer, as well. The Vermont Back Research Center at the University of Vermont in Burlington looked at a variety of anxiety provokers such as stressful marriage, job dissatisfaction, and trouble getting along with co-workers. "People who recovered from back injuries who had less of those stressors in their life tended not to have chronic pain," says Rebecca Mueller, M.A., who notes that such factors are a large part of the back pain literature today.

"Psychosocial variables are being looked at to find out which is the chicken and the egg."

"The stress relief component of back pain is the most ignored," says physiatrist Richard Materson, M.D., who levels a good part of the blame at doctors who don't spend enough time with patients to get an idea of their mental state. "If you go see a doctor who has roughly ten minutes to see you, you don't have a relationship that makes you very willing to expose yourself emotionally to that person." And all too often, the doctor might not even ask you to try.

We'll explore the mind-body connection in more detail in chapter 7. Meanwhile, here are some tips for handling immediate stress:

• **Cool down.** "The person who has the facet joint problem who doesn't experience pain when they're cool and calm, but feels it when they're mad at the boss might find that learning to get cool may in essence do more for his back pain than fixing the joint," says Dr. Materson.

• **Take some deep breaths.** Breathe in and out deeply to send nourishing oxygen through the system and relax tensed muscles.

• **Change your focus.** Turn your gaze from what's troubling you for a while; when you return, you'll often find you have a different perspective.

• **Talk it out.** Find a friend and unburden yourself. A lighter load is easier to handle.

• **Take a brisk walk.** Physical activity not only serves as a healthy diversion but brings about hormonal changes that physically fight stress.

F.Y.I.

Use progressive relaxation as a method to get yourself to relax. A simple exercise of physical release, progressive relaxation works by tensing individual muscles or muscle groups for about ten seconds at a time, and then loosening, then tensing and loosening again and again. You'll feel the body untightening and unwinding from pent-up stress.

F.Y.I.

More than 100 million Americans of all ages regularly fail to get a good night's sleep.

At least eighty-four types of disorders of sleeping and waking interfere with quality of life and personal health.

Source: American Sleep Disorders Association

When We're Tired

According to the American Sleep Disorders Association in Rochester, Minnesota, more than 100 million Americans of all ages regularly fail to get a good night's snooze. And the National Sleep Foundation in Washington, D.C., tells us that 67 percent of 1,027 Americans surveyed report sleep problems; 37 percent say they are so sleepy during the day that it interferes with their activities; and 23 percent acknowledge having fallen asleep while driving during the past year.

That means a lot of us are yawning a lot during the day, and we're more susceptible to accidents that come from not being alert, and to the impairment in general health that comes from a lack of adequate rest.

As basic as nutrition, sleep is essential to a healthy life. And the healthier we are, the less susceptible we are to injury and illness that can cause back pain. Lack of sleep lowers immunity and makes us more susceptible to physical illness. Increased irritability, clouded thinking, and physical weakness wreak havoc upon our daily life. We're less able to focus, we make more mistakes, and we are more likely to react with our emotions rather than with our heads. (And if you've already forgotten what that can do, re-read the section on stress, above.)

Without enough sleep, disease processes can be aggravated, from arthritis and other pain problems to conditions related to the autoimmune and central nervous systems to psychological disorders. Even mild sleep loss can reduce our ability to think clearly and slow our reaction time. But the amount of sleep we need varies so much from person to person, and at different stages of life, that putting a number on how many hours we should get could keep anyone tossing and turning.

"The only way to tell whether you've had enough is how you function during the day on a sustained basis," says Peter Hauri, Ph.D., of the Sleep Disorders Center at Mayo Clinic Rochester, in Minnesota. "If you are not sleepy when you watch TV at night or are sitting in a boring meeting, then you probably had enough."

While the quality of your sleep is important to your body's health, the quality of what you sleep on matters, too. In chapter 8 we look into a variety of sleep products on the market. Meanwhile, here are some hints for sound sleep:

• **Don't eat a heavy meal before bedtime.** It'll keep your body at work digesting.

• **Put a limit on or eliminate caffeine, alcohol, and tobacco consumption, especially with or after dinner.** Remember that caffeine includes soft drinks and chocolate.

• **Keep a regular sleep schedule.** Go to bed and get up at the same times every day, including weekends. Establishing regular times for meals, medications, chores, and other activities can also help.

• **Establish a pre-sleep ritual.** Try a warm bath and fifteen minutes of a soothing book (no suspense thrillers) each night. Remember: The purpose is to *wind down.*

• **Don't take "catch up" naps.** A balance of mental and physical activity throughout the day will help you sleep better at night. If you enjoy a nap, try to take it at the same time every afternoon.

• **Make your bedroom a stress-free zone.** Associate it with peace, rest, and loving intimacy with your partner. Remove tension-producing objects such as office work and required reading. When you retire for the night, keep the shades down and the television off.

• **Invest in a high-quality mattress and bedding.** You spend a lot of time in bed; don't skimp.

• **Exercise regularly.** A study reported in the *Journal of the American Medical Association* found that subjects with sleep disorders who participated in a moderate exercise program enjoyed a better overall quality of sleep, fell asleep faster, and slept longer than those who didn't exercise. But do separate your exercise routine from your sleep routine: at least six hours between a workout and bedtime with vigorous exercise and at least four hours with mild exercise.

• **Avoid sleeping pills.** If you must use them, be conservative. And *never* take them when you've consumed or will be consuming alcohol.

• **Sleep right.** "In all reality, I don't think people have any control over the way they sleep," says orthopedic surgeon David Montgomery. But at least we can start out right. In general, it's better to sleep with the hips and knees bent. If you lie on your back, put one or two pillows beneath your knees. Better yet, lie on your side with hips and knees bent, and a pillow between your knees. Under your head, a flat pillow is best.

In Which Position Do You Usually Sleep?

On your side	59%
On your back	18%
On your stomach	13%
Other	4%
Don't know/no response	6%

Source: Bruskin-Goldring Research

- **Wake right.** Just as important as how you sleep is how you wake. When you're ready to get out of bed, roll onto your side, let your legs drop off the bed and push up with your arms.

With Seasonal Hazards

Although the classic picture of back pain is that of the suburban homeowner with one hand on his lower spine and the other on a snow shovel, back care specialists report they see more people in the warmer months.

Just as sure as April showers and May flowers, the "ouch" of an aching back is a sure sign that spring has sprung. Fresh from sedentary months of winter hibernation, eager to jump into action in the great outdoors, we risk serious pain—and bodily harm.

"When spring comes around and the weather changes, a lot of people decide it's time to get out and be active after being sedentary most of the winter," says Dr. David Montgomery.

Cold-weather couch potatoes are advised to take it slow when resuming sports activities or other physical pursuits in which they haven't been involved for a while. And we're not just talking about touch football. Gardening, too, presents challenges; planting, digging, weeding, and cleaning up the yard involve a lot of lifting and bending, pushing and pulling—all activities that put a lot of strain on the back.

"A lot of people are out of shape and they all of a sudden want to start vigorous activity," says Dr. Montgomery. "A better way to approach this is to start getting in shape before spring arrives with aerobic conditioning, walking, stationary-bike rid-

Doing something we're not used to too vigorously is a sure way to give ourselves sore muscles. And with the first snowfall, or the coming of spring, we're eager to get outside and ski, shovel, or garden. "Build your spine up to it," advises Randall Braddom, M.D., medical director of Wishard Health Services in Indianapolis, and a professor at Indiana University School of Medicine. Dr. Braddom advocates following an athlete's example and increase your level of training gradually, by 10 percent increments. "Keep fit, so when you do meet a circumstance where you have to do something vigorous, you can. You never know when you're going to have to shovel snow."

ing, nonimpact aerobics, a Stairmaster—all activities that can be done indoors before spring arrives to get in shape for the mild weather."

In addition to the basics of lifting you'll find in chapter 4, here are some special changing-season tips:

- **Gear up for activity in advance with a healthy exercise routine.** Aerobic conditioning, walking, swimming, or cycling can keep your back and the muscles that support it flexible and strong.

- **Check your equipment.** Before returning to the baseball game or ski slopes after a season away, check to be sure your shoes, skis, and all other equipment is in good condition and appropriate to the sport or task at hand.

- **Support yourself all year.** When you're gardening, sit on the ground and lean on one arm to lessen back strain. When you're shoveling snow, establish a firm stance so that you won't fall; bend at the knees, not the back, and turn with your feet, not by twisting. Whatever the task or time of year, keeping your movements smart will reduce the risk of injury.

When We're Old ...
and Sedentary

Degenerative changes in the disks cause their soft nuclei to harden and become susceptible to rupture; joints become worn; and bone-weakening osteoporosis affects four in ten women over the age of seventy-five. Almost every one of us will experience wear and tear or hormone-related changes with age, but disability is not a "natural" product of aging.

"People in America don't wear out, we rust out," says Randall L. Braddom, M.D., M.S., professor of physical medicine and rehabilitation at Indiana University School of Medicine. "Elderly folks in our country tend not to be very active, and as they lose strength are more susceptible to, [for instance,] falling. All of us are always tripping all our life. If you have strength, you can catch yourself before you fall. Without strength, you have no margin for error.

"There is a tendency in our society for the elderly to be weak," Dr. Braddom continues, noting that a sixty-year-old man will have twice as much body fat and half as much muscle as a thirty-year-old of the same weight. Some is hormonal, some due to aging, he says, estimating that as much as 80 percent might be due to lack of exercise. "It's a phenomenon of disuse, not aging."

Not all of the effects of aging can be avoided, but many can be slowed. Here's some advice on how to maintain fitness as you age:

• **Stay active.** Physical exercise builds up muscles and bones whereas inactivity allows them to degenerate.

• **Stay strong.** Don't forget strength training. "We're not trying to make Charles Atlases," says Randall. "Just maintain the strength you had when younger."

• **Don't be heroic.** Use proper lifting and moving techniques (see chapter 4). And get help when you need it.

• **Watch your weight.** Extra pounds present the body with extra stress. And nutritional needs change with age; so should your diet.

• **Don't smoke.** In addition to causing other problems, smoking wreaks havoc on the circulatory system and robs the body of nutrients.

• **Sit smart.** Maintain good posture when standing and sitting.

During Pregnancy

One of the most common discomforts of pregnancy, back pain can be expected by about half of all expectant moms. Experiencing back pain before pregnancy and having had more than one pregnancy increase the risk. It might seem a wonder that more pregnant women *don't* experience back pain, what with all the musculoskeletal, weight, and hormonal changes that occur.

To accommodate a shifted center of gravity and stay upright, pregnant women must alter their posture in spine-stressing ways. Meanwhile, as the pregnancy progresses, the hormone *relaxin*, which allows the pelvis to expand for the growing baby, increases tenfold, loosening ligaments and joints, which alters balance. Abdominal muscles become stretched by the enlarging uterus, reducing their tone and their ability to keep the body in a neutral posture that doesn't stress the spine.

Pregnancy back pain is usually felt in the low back, in one or a combination of three types:

1. **Lumbar pain.** Occurring in the lower area of the spine, lumbar pain can be experienced with or

without pain in the legs. It is prompted by carrying weight or sitting for long periods. Turning in bed at night can make it feel worse.

2. Sacroiliac pain. Four times more common than lumbar pain is sacroiliac pain, which is felt lower than and on the side of the lumbar spine in the pelvis and buttocks, sometimes radiating down to knee level or beyond. Symptoms of sacroiliac joint pain, the longest-lasting, can continue for months after delivery. This type of pain can be brought on by staying in one position for a prolonged period, heavy loads, and turning in bed. It's been estimated that 20 to 30 percent of pregnant women experience both lumbar and sacroiliac pain.

3. Nocturnal pain. The third type of pain is felt only at night while lying down. Nocturnal pain is cramplike, reminiscent of the low backache of menstruation, and can wake a woman from sleep, although turning in bed won't hurt. Theories about its causes include the accumulation of the day's muscle fatigue, and circulatory slow-downs associated with lying down.

Backache of any kind can interfere with sleep and waking activity, both of which are important to a healthy pregnancy. In addition to observing standard precautions against back pain, pregnant women are advised to consider the following list of recommendations to help prevent and cope with back pain.

• **Consult your doctor.** Don't take any medications—not even over-the-counter remedies—without your physician's approval.

• **Use moderate heat and ice instead of drugs.** A warm shower or bath might ease your pain, but avoid hot water, Jacuzzis or whirlpool baths, and heating pads.

• **Watch your posture.** Physicians can teach you the neutral spine posture that avoids excessive lumbar lordosis (lower back curving), and excessive reversal of it.

• **Massage therapy may provide short-term pain relief.** Be sure to tell your massage therapist that you're pregnant, and avoid excessive joint manipulation.

• **Sleep smart.** To relieve or prevent night pain, sleep on your side, with a pillow beneath the abdomen and between the legs. Bend the lower knee and prop the other leg with a pillow. Full-body pillows and other ergonomic devices can also help during sleep and waking hours (see chapter 8).

• **Exercise appropriately.** Pregnancy-appropriate exercise programs can help relieve lumbar and sacroiliac pain. Start out with a trained physical therapist well-versed in pregnancy-related aches. Exercises that are done lying flat on the back should be modified or omitted after the first trimester.

• **No X-rays.** Radiographs are not part of the diagnostic workup for pregnant women who have back pain. An MRI can be performed if the doctor suspects a neurological cause severe enough to merit surgery or other invasive treatment.

Food for Thought . . . and Back Health

Food has a lot to do with backache, and we're not just talking about the hazard of carrying a week's worth of groceries and other necessities up the stairs. When it comes to back pain, nutrition plays a dual role: what we eat has a lot to do with how healthy our bones and muscles are, and with whether or not we are overweight. Both are important factors in back health.

Extra pounds mean extra strain on the spine and all its supportive tissues, and "overweight" or "obesity" will appear on most every back pain risk factor list.

"There's really no diet that cures back pain except insomuch as it reduces weight," says Elizabeth Ward, M.S., R.D., spokesperson for the American Dietetic Association (ADA). "If you're overweight, chances are it will aggravate your back, especially if you're carrying [the excess bulk] in your belly."

But the pain itself can slow the process of losing the extra pounds. "People in so much pain sometimes find it hard to move around enough to get or keep the weight off," adds Ward. "They become more sedentary because of the pain." The more sedentary, the less likely the weight loss, the more pain, and on and on.

A sensible diet that includes all the food groups from the USDA Food Guide Pyramid is the only sure-fire prescription, with special attention paid to particular dietary needs.

Athletes and those who exercise intensely place extra demands on their bodies, using more energy, losing more body fluid, and putting more stress on

SMART SOURCES

Center for Nutrition Policy and Promotion
1120 20th St. NW, Suite 200, North Lobby
Washington, D.C. 20036
202-606-8000
www.usda.gov/fcs/cnpp.htm

For free copies of the USDA Food Guide Pyramid and the "Dietary Guidelines for Americans," write or call this center or visit its Web site.

muscles, joints, and bones. Pregnant women have increased calcium needs. Vegans—vegetarians who do not consume any animal products at all—can usually get enough calcium, but they must watch for vitamin B_{12}, found only in meats and animal products, fortified breakfast cereals, or through vitamin supplements. (Note: Studies have found that vegetarians are able to absorb and retain more calcium from foods and have lower rates of osteoporosis than nonvegetarians. Calcium-retaining properties of soy protein, a vegetarian staple, surely help.)

The 30 to 50 million Americans who are lactose intolerant and cannot digest significant amounts of this enzyme found primarily in milk and dairy products must be vigilant to get enough calcium. But even older women at risk for osteoporosis can meet most of their special dietary needs by eating leafy greens, fish, and other lactose-free, calcium-rich foods.

For all of us, a varied, balanced eating plan that supplies the right amount of nutrients and energy is necessary to perform at our best, preventing fatigue and related injury in the process. Not only does the body need specific vitamins and minerals, but *how* we consume them can help us process the nutrients better (we can absorb only so much vitamin C at a time, for instance). Here's some sound nutrition and lifestyle advice that will also aid in maintaining back health:

• **Eat a varied, well-balanced diet.** Follow USDA Food Pyramid guidelines; don't overdo the protein; and use sodium, caffeine, and alcohol in moderation (if at all) to maximize intake of essential nutrients, and minimize risks for osteoporosis and other diseases.

- **Graze.** The latest research is leaning away from the "three squares" to a "grazing" approach: smaller meals, four to six times a day, give the body a more consistent supply of fuel. Also, by lessening the chance that we'll be "starving" before our next meal, it can help us to eat more sensibly and be less frantic about food preparation, making the meal less stressful and easier to digest.

- **Don't overdo weight-loss diets.** If you need to lose weight, be sure you don't lose out on needed nutrients. If you have a family history of osteoporosis, contact a registered dietitian to address this or other special health needs.

Crash Diets

No matter how much weight you're out to lose, crash and fad diets are not the way to lose it. Very low calorie diets backfire when your body, trying to save you from starvation, slows the metabolism (your energy-burning capacity), which slows the weight loss. And the lowered metabolic rate can continue even after you start eating normally again. This explains what happens with "yo-yo dieting," where weight is gained and lost in cycles of severely restricted diets: the metabolism falls lower and lower, and weight is harder to lose each time around.

"Miracle" diets don't work, either. And they, too, can be dangerous. Beware of regimes with an all-or-nothing approach that rely heavily on food supplements or exclude major food groups—*all* the fruits you want, *unlimited* starches, *no* protein, *no* carbohydrates, *no* fats.

To control the amount of calories coming in and to maximize your body's ability to use the calories, slow and steady weight loss of one-half to one pound a week is key. (Note: the faster you lose weight, the more likely you'll gain it back.) Cut about five hundred calories a day from your diet; eat healthy, low-fat foods; and engage in a regular exercise activity that you enjoy.

The Seven Dietary Guidelines for Good Health

The United States Department of Agriculture's Food Guide Pyramid was designed to guard against both nutritional deficiencies and consumption excesses. At the core of the pyramid's plan are the seven dietary guidelines for Americans. These guidelines for proper diet and a regular exercise regimen will go a long way to helping you maintain a healthy weight, a sure preventive measure to stave off back pain.

1. Eat a variety of foods.

2. Get plenty of vegetables, fruits, and grains.

3. Watch for fat, saturated fat, and cholesterol.

4. Use sugars in moderation.

5. Include salt sparingly.

6. Maintain a healthy weight.

7. Drink alcohol in moderation, if at all.

Source: U.S. Department of Agriculture

• **Be physically active.** Exercise does not mean just a few jumping jacks. Walk, run, dance, play tennis, participate in team sports, weight train, ride a bike; the point here is to regularly do something that you enjoy to keep yourself active.

• **Don't smoke or abuse alcohol.** Both substances are associated with a wide range of serious health hazards, from lung cancer and emphysema to kindey damage and liver disease. In addition, smoking lowers levels of bone-strengthening estrogen in the body, and alcohol can leech calcium from the blood.

Get Milk!

The calcium and vitamin D contained in milk can make a big difference in back strength.

"Absolutely necessary for bone health is calcium. Adults need at least 1,000 milligrams of calcium a day," says nutritionist Elizabeth Ward. "The thing about drinking milk is that it also provides vitamin D, which is needed to absorb the calcium into the body, and milk is among the only foods that's fortified with vitamin D."

If you think of the bones as the body's calcium bank account, suggests Ward, vitamin D is the bank teller, doling out proper amounts of calcium to keep levels constant in the bloodstream. If we don't get enough calcium in the food we eat, the body withdraws it from the bones. Years of chronic deprivation will leave the bones bankrupt. Here's some bone-solid advice:

- **Get your daily requirement.** Up to the age of fifty, says Ward, we need 200 IUs (International Units) of calcium a day. Between the ages of fifty-one and seventy, we need 400 IUs, and after that, 600 IUs per day. The ADA recommends general calcium intake of 1,500 milligrams daily to reduce bone loss in later years. Three or more servings of calcium-rich foods (non- and low-fat yogurt, milk, and other dairy products, as well as spinach and certain fruits) are a good start.

- **Beware of "calcium leeches."** High-salt, high-protein diets exhaust the body's supply of calcium, as does alcohol and certain medications, such as prednisone. If you're taking medication, ask your doctor or pharmacist about *all* its effects and compensate where necessary.

- **Think twice about protein.** Whether or not protein-rich diets prompt the loss of body calcium and contribute to osteoporosis is under debate. Recent studies dispute the belief, saying that it originated in earlier studies based on pure protein, which does not contain calcium-saving phosphorus or other nutrients found in meat, fish, and poultry that may counterbalance the protein's effects. Stay tuned.

- **Meet your needs for vitamin D.** Moderate amounts of sunlight and a proper diet are both good sources: enjoy fifteen minutes out in the sun at least three or more times weekly, and include vi-

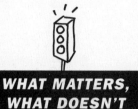

WHAT MATTERS, WHAT DOESN'T

What Matters

- Being aware of the many possible causes of back pain so that you can remedy those you already have and prevent others.

- Knowing when you're most susceptible to back pain so that you can be more vigilant at those times.

- Maintaining a healthy diet to keep your back—and the rest of your body—in good health.

What Doesn't

- Knowing the many possible causes of back pain, and when you're more susceptible, if you do nothing about them.

- Your age alone. Lifestyle has a great deal to do with susceptibility to back pain.

- A reliance on nutritional supplements without regard for the needed foods.

tamin D–rich foods (milk, breakfast cereals, beef liver, salmon, mackerel) in meals you prepare.

A sound diet and prepared mind go a long way toward preventing or remedying much back pain. Proper physical movement goes further still. The next chapter explores how.

THE BOTTOM LINE

The list of possible causes of back pain is a long one, but a general familiarity with the problems, from serious maladies to temporary setbacks due to life changes, and with their warning signs can provide helpful clues to both cure and prevention. Knowing when we're most susceptible can keep us alert and safer, and recognizing the valuable role of nutrition can keep us healthy and strong.

Form, Movement, and Exercise

Looking on the bright side, the fact that so many back problems are self-inflicted can give us cause to rejoice. If they are self-inflicted, after all, that means we have at least a chance of stopping them from happening to us. The effect of bad habits in the way we move—and stay still—can be felt immediately, or build up over weeks, months, even years. The good news is that they can be corrected by good posture and the right exercise.

Good Form

Even when we're not moving—sometimes *because* we're not—we are exerting pressure and stress on our backs. Alf L. Nachemson, M.D., Ph.D., a Swedish orthopedic surgeon, is world-renowned for his research on the spine and his findings related to the amount of pressure exerted on the disks when we are in different positions.

"Measurements of pressure over the last twenty years in more than one hundred individuals have demonstrated how the load on the lumbar disk varies with the position of the subject's body, and during the performance of various tasks, both in standing and in sitting," he notes in one study, published in *Spine* magazine. "Compared with the pressure of load in the upright standing position, reclining reduces the pressure by 50 to 80 percent, while unsupported sitting increases the load by 40 percent, forward leaning and weight lifting by more than 100 percent, and the position of forward flexion and rotation by 400 percent."

In other words, sitting is more stressful to our backs than standing, leaning forward is worse, and twisting worse still. And whatever position we're in, poor posture exacerbates the problem.

There is a better way. In fact, there are many of them. Here, some of the best:

While You're Sitting

• **Know how you got there.** To get into a chair, bend your knees and lower yourself onto its front edge, then scoot back. To get up, reverse the process by placing one foot forward and moving to the front of the seat. Use a rocking motion to stand.

• **Don't slouch.** Slouching—with its characteristic hunched back and shoulders—overstretches muscles and ligaments, yet it is our natural tendency as our back muscles get tired, especially in a chair that doesn't provide proper support. Stay in touch with your posture, and readjust.

• **Sit back for support.** Whatever it is that keeps you on the edge of your seat will keep your back from feeling its best. Keep the small of your back against the back rest. If the chair doesn't provide sufficient support (or is too deep to allow your knees to bend over the front edge when you're in it), place a lumbar cushion, pillow or rolled towel at the small of your back.

• **Make adjustments.** Many office chairs allow adjustments to be made to height, seat, back, tilt, even armrests. For desk work that calls for upright sitting, knees should be level with or slightly lower than the level of your hips. Arm rests should allow you to comfortably rest your forearms with your el-

SMART MOVE

If your boss won't spring for a new, adjustable chair (even after you've told him of the costs of the nation's back pain–related workers, compensation claims), less expensive alternatives might work. "If the seat is too deep, put [an office-chair-appropriate] lumbar cushion behind you—it will fill the space and give lumbar support," suggests ergonomics consultant Ira Janowitz, at the University of California. If arm rests are the problem, check to see whether those on your current chair are removable, or if the chair allows new rests to be put on. Velcro-attachable pads can raise their height or soften them.

The Three Kinds of Sitting

1. Upright sitting. Good for keyboard use, this posture is the one to which most people are referring when they say "sit." Thighs are at right angles to the trunk, which is in a vertical position; the head is balanced over the shoulders. On the downside: increased pressure on lumbar disks.

2. Forward sitting. The position we automatically take to read material that's on our desktop. Knees drop lower than hip level, and the trunk inclines forward. Chairs with forward-tilting seats can help keep us from a Quasimodo-level "hunch."

3. Reclining. Not just for La-Z-Boys, this is a nice alternative posture for talking on the phone or taking in a good book. In the right chair, the hips don't have to scoot forward, and the back is well-supported. Reclining takes weight off the upper body and relieves pressure on lumbar disks.

bows bent more or less at right angles, and shoulders relaxed, without interfering with the tasks at hand.

- **Feet flat on the floor.** If your feet can't reach the floor and your chair isn't adjustable, foot rests are an often-recommended option. That may be fine if you're putting up your feet for an extended period, but if you're at the office, a footrest can discourage movement and may prompt you to twist as you reach for the phone or fax. You can also trip over it. A better solution, if possible, is to build a low platform into the space beneath the desk.

- **Change postures.** Even if you must stay seated all day, it doesn't mean you can't change positions (see the box above).

• **Get up and go.** The best way to avoid the risks of sitting for prolonged periods is not to do it. Take frequent short breaks—at least one every twenty to thirty minutes—to stand up and stretch.

While You're Standing

• **Shift positions frequently.** As with sitting, standing for extended periods of time causes the back muscles to relax, causing our posture to sag, which stresses the spine. As you notice this happening, straighten: keep your chest up, stomach in, and buttocks tightened.

• **Rest one foot on a low stool or shelf.** Ever wonder why the bar rail came to be? Bartenders discovered that their standing patrons will drink longer if they're comfortable. Alternate the elevated foot periodically.

• **Don't stoop over.** If you must remain standing for long periods while you work—and that includes dusting and ironing—keep your work close to you and at a comfortable height so that you don't have to bend over to see or do it. Otherwise, bend your knees, kneel, or sit. If stooping is unavoidable, take regular breaks to stand upright and stretch backward.

• **Wear sensible shoes.** High heels are a health hazard. Not only do they throw the body out of alignment, causing the low back to arch excessively and increasing stress, but they increase the likelihood of a fall. Pointy-toed shoes, too, can prompt an unhealthy distribution of your weight. Wear comfortable, low-heeled shoes with good arch supports.

While You're Lying Down

• **Sleep right.** As we mentioned earlier, we have only so much control over the position in which we sleep (see chapter 3 for the positions most recommend—on the side or back). If you must sleep on your stomach, elevate your lower legs (and stomach or chest, if needed) with a good-size pillow. Lumbar rolls can provide support to the lower back no matter how much we roll around, but can take some getting used to. (More about this and other posture aids in chapter 8.)

• **Check your mattress.** Most back problems that result from sleep posture stem from a worn or inappropriate (too soft *or* too hard) mattress. If yours is over ten years old, or sags, go directly to chapter 8.

• **"Get there" right.** Sit on the side of the bed, and lower yourself onto your side by raising your legs and lowering your head at the same time, using your arms to keep you from twisting. Bend both knees to roll onto your back, if desired. To sit up, reverse the process. If you find this difficult, try getting into bed on hands and knees before lowering yourself; reverse the process to get up.

• **Enjoy a morning stretch.** You may have awakened, but your muscles are still at rest. Slowly stretch before rising, and again once you get out of bed.

• **Recline right.** If you spend a fair amount of time reclining on the sofa, or if you're fond of putting your feet up on the coffee table while you're sitting in an armchair, do it right—supporting, not twisting or suspending your back in a position from which you'll have to strain to rise.

Good Moves

By now you know that the most common type of back pain comes from straining the muscles surrounding the spine. The lumbar area—the curve of the low back—is the most common site of pain and injury. Not only does it support the most body weight, but it bears the bulk of the strain involved in sitting, bending and—what so often puts us at risk—lifting. The second most popular trouble spot is the base of the neck.

Moving the wrong way can hurt. "Inappropriate body mechanics are probably the most lethal [risk to the back]," says physical therapist Elaine R. Rosen, P.T., M.S., D.P.T., O.C.S., of Hunter College, City University of New York. "You don't need to lift a lot of weight or do something excessive, it's *how* you do it."

Being in good physical shape can reduce the risk, and the exercises in the section beginning on page 104 can help. But even the strongest and most flexible among us will benefit from using the right techniques.

Bending

• **Try not to do it.** Bending at the waist and rising on the power of the spine is one of the major causes of back trouble. Opt to squat, kneel, or sit. Whatever you choose, keep the pressure off your back. When you garden, sit on the ground and lean on one arm; when you put on your socks, keep your back straight and bend your legs; when you reach into your car trunk, place one foot on the bumper and slide items close before lifting. Another helpful trick: keep your back straight and lift one leg backward while using the opposite hand for support—helpful for many "deep reaches," such as into a washing machine or grocery cart.

• **But if you must bend . . .** If you're caring for a baby or tending someone confined to bed, try your best to sit or stand with your knees bent and your back straight. If you absolutely cannot, be sure to stand straight at frequent intervals and take a stretching (bending backward) break.

Lifting and Carrying

• **Warm up to the task.** Before lifting anything (and afterward, too), perform some stretching movements to limber up.

• **Stay balanced.** Plant your feet at least shoulder-width apart for a solid base of support.

• **Keep your back straight and don't twist.** Use the strength of your legs, not your spine. Bend at the knees, not at the waist, and to get up push off on one foot if necessary. A back support such as those worn by the salespeople at many home-supply stores can keep you from bending at the waist, but some believe long-term use can lead to weaker back muscles.

• **Stay close.** Never lift anything with your arms extended. Before the lift, get as close to the object as you can; the nearer it is, the less stress on the back. Heavy objects are best carried at waist or pelvis level, no higher. "Carry heavy things at the center of gravity of the body or as close as possible," says Randall L. Braddom, M.D., M.S., of the Indiana University School of Medicine. "The center of gravity is two centimeters in front of the second sacral vertebra—where God, in her wisdom, put the uterus. That's a good place to carry things."

• **Don't reach.** On the same principle as above, once you have lifted something, don't extend your arms with the object in them. According to Dr. Nachemson's studies, holding five kilograms (eleven pounds) with your arms extended exerts more pressure than lifting twice as much with your back straight and your knees bent. Walk over close to where you are taking the object and use a step-stool to reach anything above shoulder height.

• **Push, don't pull.** It exerts less pressure. Keep your back properly aligned and use leg muscles to do the work.

• **Know your load.** Trouble can result when there's a mismatch between the amount of weight you think you're picking up and what you actually are—and heavy objects aren't the only ones that present a risk. Gearing up to lift a heavy suitcase and abruptly finding out it's empty, for instance, will result in a more extreme and sudden movement than that for which you were prepared. It's called unexpected load. Your brain calculates what the load is going to be and readies the muscles accordingly, and if it gets surprised you can get a strain or a sprain. "Test" the load first.

SMART DEFINITION

Ergonomics

The science of fitting the job to the worker. When there is a mismatch between the physical requirements of the job and the physical capacity of the worker, work-related musculoskeletal disorders (WMSDs) can result. Workers who must repeat the same motion throughout their workday, who must do their work in an awkward position, who must use a great deal of force to perform their jobs, who must repeatedly lift heavy objects, or who face a combination of these risk factors are most likely to develop WMSDs.

Source: Occupational Safety and Health Administration

• **Brace yourself.** For heavier objects, keep your abdominal muscles braced, but don't hold your breath.

• **Even out.** Try to balance the weight evenly. Instead of one heavy suitcase, pack two lighter ones, and carry one in each hand. If you must tote a heavy purse or bookbag, don't lug it all on one shoulder; opt for a backpack that evenly distributes the weight.

• **Get help.** Don't try to lift objects that are too heavy or awkward to grasp. The right tool, dolly, wheelbarrow, or friend can lighten your load.

Turning

• **Don't twist your spine.** Turn or pivot the whole body in the direction you want to move—feet first.

At the Office

Is the desk at which you spend eight hours a day so high or wide that you have to strain to reach objects at its far edge? Does your telephone feel like a permanent connection linking your shoulder to your ear? Is the dimness of your computer display keeping your face so close to the monitor that your neck is permanently crooked?

Ergonomics takes all these factors into account. "People in this country tend to think of ergonomics as body posture and position, maybe movement, but not in terms of the total environment," says Ira L. Janowitz, P.T., C.P.E., of the University of California Ergonomics Program. "That is just a small part of it," says Janowitz, who defines the science as the study of the relationship of people to their work and work environment.

Ventilation, office stress, the carpet beneath your swivel chair—anything that affects the relationship between you and your work can concern an ergonomist . . . and your back. An ergonomist would consider whether the lighting is too dim to allow for safety or whether deadline pressure keeps you from taking occasional breaks.

In "Tips for Healthy Computer Use," on the University of California Ergonomics Program Web site, director David M. Rempel, M.D., emphasizes three points that can be applied to computer work or any kind of desk work: *Position* your equipment properly, *relax* your shoulders and hands while working, and *vary* your workday.

"Think about adjusting everything to find your most effective body postures for your most common tasks," writes Dr. Rempel. "In general, you should adjust your chair first, your keyboard and mouse second, and your monitor and print material third."

Whether your day is spent on the computer, the telephone, or over hard copy, several desk strategies can reduce the possibility of injury to or strain of your back.

• **Sit right.** Follow the strategies outlined earlier in this chapter.

• **Keep tools close.** Arrange your work area so that frequently used items are within easy reach.

• **Consider a headset.** If you spend significant amounts of time on the telephone—especially

SMART MOVE

As important as it is, education alone will not prevent back injury, emphasizes physical therapist Charles Curry, coordinator of the Musculoskeletal Injury Prevention Program at Cornell University. "People say, 'Let's teach people how to take care of their backs.' You end up with well-informed [but nevertheless injured] patients. If people learn all these things, but don't change the things that are going to hurt them, they'll have injuries at the same rate."

while you are typing—use a headset. *Do not* keep the receiver clamped to your shoulder by means of your ear.

• **Look with your eyes, not your neck.** Place whatever you look at most (either the computer screen or paperwork) directly in front of you to eliminate the need to turn your head to the side while you type. A variety of document holders on the market can hold papers at eye level.

• **Arrange your computer components.** Place the keyboard and mouse next to each other, in front of and close to you, and low enough so that you don't need to elevate your shoulders when you use them. Set up your monitor so that the top of the screen is at or slightly below eye level.

• **Type appropriately.** In general, keep your elbows at your sides and forearms parallel to the floor, resting on forearm supports, or with your upper arms hanging comfortably at your sides. But not everyone does the same sort of typing: Some, such as transcribers, who type steadily, are best served by the "floating hand" technique, with hands "floating" above the keyboard, wrists straight, shoulders relaxed, and torso in an upright or forward sitting posture. Others, such as those accessing a database or thinking out a memo, use the keyboard in small bursts, with frequent pauses. For them, forearm support is useful.

• **Soothe office stress.** No matter how well your work area is arranged, stressful office conditions—and that includes eye strain as well as your boss's temper—can cause muscles to tense. Try to become aware of the signs of stress, do what you can to remedy the causes, and put relaxation strategies to use.

Diversify the Day

"When we talk about back problems, in general, it's useful to take an anthropological approach," says ergonomist Janowitz. "The human body evolved over the past four million years in the context of the hunter-gatherer society, in which work is varied and human beings perform a variety of activities, as opposed to our society, where people tend to maintain static postures for prolonged periods of time. In the office, it's sitting; at an assembly line it's a static standing posture. Our ancestors didn't stand or sit for eight hours at a time—they'd walk, pick up a baby, hunt, pick berries. We're well adapted to that, changing position frequently.

"We're well designed for the upright posture. We're not well designed for the repetitive tasks and static positions of agriculture, industry, and the office. Those run counter to how the human body is 'designed' to function." "Variety is the spice of life"; it is also key to back health.

• **Vary tasks throughout the day.** Include activities that force you to change your position: stand up, lean back, walk around, climb some stairs. Do some filing, go to the copy machine, do anything that involves walking, standing, and stretching.

• **Change your posture.** Change from sitting, to standing, to sitting whenever possible. "Desk jockeys" can set aside a surface, such as a podium or a standing desk, at a comfortable standing height (about elbow level) to do some reading, for in-

F.Y.I.

Putting on the Pressure

Approximate load on the lumbar 3 disk in a person weighing 154 pounds:

Position	Units of Pressure on a Lumbar Disk
Lying down	250
Standing	500
Sitting upright	700

Source: "Disc Pressure Measurements," A. L. Nachemson, *Spine,* 1981 Jan.–Feb.; 6(1):93–7.

stance. Another excellent strategy is to put the phone near that surface and, whenever it rings, take that as a cue to stand. Remember, too, the strategies discussed earlier in this chapter—there's more than one way to sit or stand.

- **Take frequent, short breaks.** In terms of your back, they're far more helpful (in many ways) than two-hour lunches. Every twenty to thirty minutes, get up and stretch muscles and joints that were in one position for an extended period of time; relax those that were active. Use a timer so you won't forget.

"People have to listen to their bodies, and respond appropriately," says Janowitz. "Don't just follow the rules." If a chair seat is too deep for you, put a cushion behind your back; if you wear bifocals, a lower screen height might prevent you from craning your neck. Most ergonomists recommend keeping your feet flat on the floor or on a footstool, but Janowitz says: "If your feet are more comfortable on the base of the chair, fine. It's got to fit your body. We're not talking about robots."

If you notice that the changes in your workstation help alleviate your aches and pains, you've done well. But if you feel worse, don't give up. Try something else.

"Whatever strategies you use have to not only fit your body but the task and the job demands that you have to do," says Janowitz. "The same chair that is fine for a receptionist is not going to be fine for a lawyer who's going to be reading for long periods in a reclining position. We have to be job specific and take into account the particular needs of that person in the context of their job."

On the Road

We've already reviewed the impact prolonged sitting can have on your back. Add to that the vibration of the road, the stress of rush-hour traffic, and a few potholes and Sunday drivers, and you've got a backache waiting to happen.

In addition to the guidelines for proper sitting on pages 91–92, drivers and passengers can benefit from these car-specific tips.

• **Sit, then swing.** With your back to the car seat, sit down first, then swing your legs into the car, one at a time. Once you're settled, adjust yourself properly in the seat. When entering a truck or more highly elevated sport utility vehicle, use the step-up or running board.

• **Adjust your seat and wheel.** Position yourself so your knees are slightly bent when your foot is on the pedal and your elbows are comfortably bent when your hands are on the wheel. The back of the seat should be slightly reclined, and the head rests adjusted to your carmaker's specifications.

• **Adjust rear- and side-view mirrors for optimal visibility.** If you have to look back over your shoulder, do so carefully, turning your body instead of twisting your head.

• **Get adequate low back support.** If necessary, use automobile-appropriate lumbar supports (see chapter 8), or place a rolled towel or cushion in the small of your back.

• **Don't overlook the scenic points of interest.** Truck drivers, who sit for lengthy drives while being jostled by vibration, lead almost all occupations in back injuries. On long trips, stop frequently to get out of the car and stretch. Not only will you relieve the pressure of prolonged sitting and benefit from a break from the vibration, but the sights (if really scenic) can reduce stress.

• **Avoid tight side-by-side parking spaces.** Squeezing out of your door sardine-style can result in risky twisting.

• **Buckle up.** If an accident happens, a seat belt can save your back . . . and your life.

Work It Out: Exercise!

How do we sprain and strain our backs? Most of the time, we hurt our backs by using them the wrong way, and/or not keeping them in good condition. In the last section of this chapter we learned how to use the back the right way via proper posture and the correct "body mechanics" of everyday movement. Here we take a look at getting it into good all-around shape.

Neither this book nor most any other source of back care information can emphasize it enough: Regular physical activity is crucial to keeping the muscles that support the back strong and flexible. It's also just about the only tried-and-true healthy way to control weight and lower the risks too many extra pounds can bring. And it even helps build strong bones.

Yet many of us just can't seem to get enough physical activity to keep in shape.

"The problem in our society is we have cars and push-button everything," says physiatrist Randall Braddom. "We drive one block, use elevators." We ride lawnmowers and golf carts, let machines wash our dishes, we don't even have to open doors ourselves. "It's the 'If you don't use it, you lose it' phenomenon. In our society it's actually possible to just atrophy."

And so, along came the high-powered gym and structured exercise. In Braddom's words: "The catch-22 of our society is that we've now gone to using exercise machines to give us back all the exercise that machines have taken away from us."

But tread carefully—especially if you're recovering from a bout with back pain—not only because you might not know what the exact problem is and what movements are safe to perform (or how many, or when) but because even the same problem might call for different exercises depending on the way in which it manifests. The best exercises if you have a bulging or herniated disk, for instance, would depend on the position in which the disk is bulging or herniated.

"It depends on what the problem is for the patient and what's causing the pain," says physical therapist Elaine Rosen. "Sometimes extension—bending backward—is best, sometimes the opposite is better. If you hand out a sheet of paper and say these are terrific exercises for everybody, you run into trouble because some people do better with one protocol and some with another."

"You really should exercise under appropriate guidance, at least initially, to start off on the right track," she cautions. "You can create a back problem with inappropriate exercise—too much, or too intense, or done incorrectly—and exacerbate an already existing problem."

SMART MOVE

Don't ignore your back pain, says Louis Kuritzky, M.D., of the University of Florida. Even though the vast majority of cases heal themselves, it can be a symptom of a much more serious problem. Aortic aneurysms, for instance, bulges or tears in the wall of the body's main artery, are commonly misdiagnosed, even when symptoms—including abdominal pain and tenderness, and back pain, suggest that a rupture might already have occured. "If you're over fifty or under twenty with new-onset back pain," says Kuritzky, "have a full evaluation, not just Motrin, rest, and a heating pad."

Prescreening for Exercise

Any reputable fitness plan will advise you to contact your doctor before you begin. In most cases, the health risks of inactivity far outweigh the risks of an exercise program, but extreme or sudden physical activity, or exercise done incorrectly, can cause musculoskeletal injury, among other hazards. And if you are starting a program because you've already hurt your back, there is special cause for moderation.

In most cases, commonsense caution and a self-administered questionnaire can help gauge readiness for a low to moderate intensity exercise program. The President's Council on Physical Fitness and Sports recommends the Revised Physical Activity Readiness Questionnaire (rPAR-Q, printed on the following page), developed in Canada and widely accepted for use in the United States, for determining exercise readiness in "symptom-free adults with no more than one major cardiac risk factor"—such as smoking, or overly high alcohol, caffeine, or drug use; high blood pressure or cholesterol levels; or overweight. Those who answer any of the questions "yes" are advised to check with a doctor first.

Some people, such as those past their mid- to late-sixties, and anyone who has been diagnosed with heart disease, arthritis, diabetes, or respiratory ailments; or anyone who has allergies, leg cramping, or feels pain upon exertion, shouldn't need the test to know a doctor's consultation is in order. The same for anyone who is pregnant or has a family history of sudden death at a young age. And if you have a cold, flu, or just don't feel well, don't exercise until you feel better.

Revised Physical Activity Readiness Questionnaire (rPAR-Q)

If you answer "no" to all of the following questions, you can be pretty sure that you can start becoming much more physically active—starting slowly and building up gradually. If you answer "yes" to one or more questions, talk with your doctor first. Answering yes doesn't mean you shouldn't increase your physical activity or that you won't benefit from it, only that you might have to avoid certain types of exercise or should start off at a slower pace. By being aware of specific areas of risk, you can be more alert to warning signs.

1. Has a doctor said that you have a heart condition and recommended only medically supervised activity?

2. Do you have chest pain brought on by physical activity?

3. Have you developed chest pain in the past month?

4. Do you tend to lose consciousness or fall over as a result of dizziness?

5. Do you have a bone or joint that could be aggravated by the proposed physical activity?

6. Has a doctor ever recommended medication for your blood pressure or a heart condition?

7. Are you aware through your own experience, or a doctor's advice, of any other physical reason against your exercising without medical supervision?

If you've begun a fitness program to relieve back pain, don't stop when the pain subsides. It's what brings clients back to the physical therapist's office time and again. "The majority of patients start to feel better, then don't do anything," says orthopedic specialist Elaine Rosen. "Their reason: 'I was doing better and felt I was cured.' I hear it all the time."

Exercise to Prevent Back Pain

In general, a well-rounded, overall fitness program is your best bet for reducing the risk of back pain. The more fit you are, the more fit your back, and the less likely it is to be injured. A well-balanced routine will increase your endurance, strength, and flexibility—all factors in maintaining a healthy back. Indeed, the American Physical Therapy Association reports that recent studies indicate that general conditioning—not the power of back muscles alone—may be the most important factor in avoiding back injury.

"Exercise can also be helpful in building and maintaining strong bones," reports the National Osteoporosis Foundation (NOF). "Exercise that forces you to work against gravity—so-called weight-bearing exercises such as walking or jogging—are beneficial. Other weight-bearing exercises include racquet sports, hiking, aerobic dance, and stair climbing." (Note: Extreme exercise that results in the cessation of menstruation in women will lead to *decreased* bone mass.)

And yes, most people with osteoporosis should exercise. "You should speak with your doctor or ask for a referral to a specialist in physical medicine to learn what type of exercises you can do safely," advises NOF, "not only to preserve bone, but also to strengthen your back and hips and maintain flexibility."

Remember what we said about the effect of emotional stress on muscle tension? Exercise can help in that department, as well. In addition to the considerable reduction in stress that comes from having a healthier, more fit body, physical activity is one of the best direct antidotes to anxiety.

Exercise stimulates chemicals called neurotransmitters, which are produced in the brain and are believed to mediate moods and emotions. In the lab, clinicians have found exercise to prompt decreases in the electrical activity of tensed muscles in people with nervous tension. They were less jittery and hyperactive. Exercise, in other words, basically provides a physical outlet for the bottled-up anxieties of life. With even a moderate physical workout, we can literally work the anxiety, the anger, and the stress out of our system.

Aerobic exercise, such as jogging or biking, that gets the heart going is the most widely touted for stress relief, but it isn't the only kind that helps. Stretching exercises and strength or resistance training, such as weight lifting or pushups, play a role as well: involving more focus than aerobics, these types of limbering exercises can increase your awareness of the individual parts of your body and help you bring them under control.

A well-balanced fitness program cannot possibly fit into one chapter of one book, but here are some tips with which to start.

• **Get help.** Especially if you've experienced back pain, be sure to follow the advice of knowledgeable professionals. "You need somebody to give you feedback as to whether you're doing it correctly or not," says physical therapist Kim Dunleavy, M.S., M.O.M.T., P.T., O.C.S., an orthopedic specialist based in Warren, Michigan. "Someone to start you off, to go through the correct methods of moving, the correct methods of stretching, the correct methods of lifting, the strengthening programs. . . . There's a fine line between the sensation that you get from working the muscle to its maximum, and when you're doing damage. And sometimes people just need to learn what that difference is so they can monitor their programs themselves."

• **Don't replace professionals' fitness instructions with do-it-yourself programs.** Supplementing your fitness knowledge with good exercise manuals and instructional videos is a good idea. But when starting out, let the experts show you the right way.

• **Start slow.** Don't begin a rigorous exercise program all at once, especially if you've been basically sedentary until now. Increasing the physical activity in your life by even moderate amounts—taking the stairs instead of the elevator, parking your car farther away and walking more—will make a difference.

• **Balance your fitness program.** Include aerobic activity for your heart and body composition; strength training to build muscle strength and endurance; and stretching exercises to increase your range of motion and lower your risk of injury while you're at work on the other two types of exercise. Overenthusiastic exercisers with an unbalanced program can end up strengthening one area of the body at the expense of another. "These are people who, in their mind, are doing the right thing," says Bill Boissonnault, M.S., P.T., president of the American Physical Therapy Association Orthopaedic Section. "They're going to exercise classes and working out, and their intentions are good, but they end up causing problems."

• **Just do something.** The best exercise is the one you will *do,* whether it's walking on a treadmill at a gym, taking a tour of the neighborhood, lifting barbells, or doing floor exercise. Whatever you choose, do it sensibly, with a balanced, personal program that suits your needs.

• **Take activity breaks during the day.** Several ten-minute exercise breaks throughout the day can be as beneficial as one longer workout.

• **Play.** Tennis, racquetball, volleyball and other active games count as exercise. And they're fun!

• **Warm up, wind down.** Always precede and follow exercise with some good, slow stretches, and a low-level version of the activity to rehearse and cool down the muscles used.

Basic Prevention

If you are a healthy, active adult, and your daily schedule keeps you on the move, you may not need a specialized exercise routine. If not, you'll benefit from a program focusing on strengthening and stretching the muscles that keep your back strong, as well as those that help support its work. The abdominal muscles, for instance, keep the spine stabilized; the large muscles of hip and thigh (the gluteals, quadriceps, and hamstrings) help perform lifting tasks; and a flexible spine, shoulders, and pelvis allow the normal curves of the spine to be maintained.

There are many exercises to condition the muscles of your body and back—be sure to use only those that are appropriate for you. Start slowly, move slowly, and gradually increase the repetitions only once you feel comfortable with the effort involved. (In addition, see "The McKenzie Exercises" box on pages 116–117.)

STREET SMARTS

"When my back went out I could have sworn I'd never be able to move again, much less exercise," remembers Mel, a textile salesman from New York City. "The problem was I thought exercising meant running the marathon. Once I was able to recover just a small amount of mobility, a physical therapist showed me some slow and easy movements that really helped."

Pelvic Tilt

Lie on your back with legs together, knees bent, feet flat on the floor, and your arms above your head. Push the small of your back flat to the floor, simultaneously tightening your abdominal muscles and buttocks. Hold for five seconds and relax. Repeat five times.

Single-Leg Raise

Lie on your back with legs together, knees bent, feet flat on the floor, and your arms above your head. Slowly raise one leg while straightening it, raising it as far as possible. Hold for five seconds, and slowly bend your knee and return to starting position. Repeat five times with each leg.

Half Sit-Up

Lie on your back with legs together, knees bent, feet flat on the floor, and your arms crossed over your chest. Slowly raise your head and shoulders. Continue raising, stretching your hands to your knees. Hold for five seconds, and then slowly return to the starting position. Repeat five times. For a variation, when your head and shoulders are up, stretch your right shoulder toward your left knee, and hold for five seconds. Then reverse. To intensify the exercise, keep your hands above your head.

Straight Back Bend

Stand with your feet about six inches apart, arms to your side. Keeping your back straight, bend your knees and hips until your thighs are parallel to the floor. Hold for five seconds, return to standing position. Repeat five times.

Hamstring Stretch

Sit on the floor, legs straight out in front of you with toes up, heels no more than six inches apart. Bend forward, slowly reaching for your toes. Hold forward position for five seconds, and slowly return to the starting position. Repeat five times.

Quadriceps Stretch

Stand straight, with the palm of your right hand on a wall or the back of a chair for balance. Grasp your left ankle with your left hand, and gently pull it back and up. Hold five seconds. Relax. Repeat three times with each leg. If you need to, use a folded towel to "lasso" your ankle.

Back Rest

Lie flat on your back, with the lower half of your legs on a chair so that your lower legs form a right angle with your thighs, which are at a right angle to your trunk. Remain for ten minutes.

Exercise with Back Pain?

Depending on the cause of your back pain, gentle exercise to improve flexibility is often among the first steps toward recovery. Only once the pain is gone or has eased sufficiently should strengthening exercises begin.

Again, we want to emphasize the importance of knowing the right techniques to apply to your particular problem. Some conditions benefit from forward bends, others are eased by leaning over backward, while still others call for exercise in a neutral stance.

SMART SOURCES

The McKenzie Institute,
  USA
600 E. Genesee St.,
  Suite 124
Syracuse, NY 13202
800-635-8380
315-471-7612
www.mckenziemdt.org

The McKenzie Institute,
  Canada
370 Fairway Garden
Newmarket, Ontario
Canada L3X 1B6
800-463-8568
905-836-8977
www.mckenziemdt.org

An international not-for-profit organization, the McKenzie Institute offers a method recommended for common back and neck problems worldwide. Call or write for a brochure or referral to a local certified practitioner. If you visit the Web site, click on the American flag for the greatest amount of general information about the approach.

The McKenzie Method—an exercise approach developed by New Zealand physiotherapist Robin McKenzie and taught at branches of the McKenzie Institute worldwide—has gained an enthusiastic following among back pain sufferers over the past few decades. One of if not the most preferred method of treatment among physical therapists today, the McKenzie philosophy "promotes the body's potential to heal itself without medication, heat, cold, ultrasound, needles, or a force introduced by the practitioner." Trained professionals work to develop the patient's self-treatment skills, in great part through physical movement and exercise.

"The ideal situation is for the patient to be able to recover without the therapist having to put their hands on the patient," says Robert L. Medcalf, P.T., Dip.MDT, a certified practitioner and teacher of the technique. "McKenzie would say the patient put their back 'out' by performing certain movements or getting into certain positions, and, in many cases, we should be able to teach the patient to put their back 'in,' so to speak, by utilizing other movements and positions identified during the examination process."

Seven basic exercises make up the exercise program, with the purpose not to strengthen the back but to abolish pain and, "where appropriate," restore normal range of motion. To determine whether the exercises are helping, the patient is exhorted to closely observe any changes in the intensity or location of the pain. Even if you don't use McKenzie's exercises, monitoring your progress is always good advice.

"If your pain moves to the midline of the spine and away from areas where it is usually felt [a phenomenon called *centralization*], you are exercising correctly and this exercise program is the correct one for you," McKenzie writes in *Treat Your Own Back,* calling centralization "the single most important guide you have in determining the correct exercise for your problem." Alternatively, if your pain moves away from the low back or increases in the buttock or leg, you are on the wrong track. Another warning sign: pain that continues to increase in intensity after the initial exercise session. Although "new" pains often temporarily develop whenever we move in ways we are not used to, they should soon subside. If any of these occur, or you notice any tingling, numbness, or any of the other "red flags" we reviewed in chapter 2, stop performing the new movements and contact a health care professional.

Look for a practitioner who is certified in the philosophies and treatments known formally as the McKenzie Method of Mechanical Diagnosis and Therapy. To qualify for the full certification program and credentialing exam, an applicant must first have obtained their credentials as a physical therapist, osteopath, chiropractor, or M.D. Look for the designation of either Cert.MDT or the more advanced Dip.MDT (Diploma in Mechanical Diagnosis and Therapy).

The Bed Rest Myth

"Two generations of people have grown up hearing that bed rest is best," says Louis Kuritzky, M.D., at the University of Florida in Gainesville's department of community health and family medicine. "But in general, the people who stay up and around are the ones who do the best."

Not even patients with sciatica, for which bed

The McKenzie Exercises

The seven main exercises of the McKenzie Method, used to eliminate back pain and to restore range of motion, are briefly described here, starting with the three "first aid" techniques for acute low back pain. Each exercise is prescribed for a particular stage in the level of pain and recovery, but all exercises should be discontinued if any of the warning signs or other pain is experienced. Sometimes other movements and guidance by a credentialed practitioner are required to benefit from the approach. For a thorough description of the exercises, and important guidelines regarding the program, contact the McKenzie Institute (see page 114) or a certified practitioner.

- **Exercise 1: Lying Face Down.** Lying face down with your arms beside your body and your head turned to one side, take a few deep breaths and relax completely for two or three minutes, making a conscious effort to remove all tension from the muscles in your low back. Used mainly in the treatment of acute back pain, this is a "first-aid exercise," and should be done once at the start of exercise sessions spread evenly six to eight times throughout the day.

- **Exercise 2: Lying Face Down in Extension.** Lying on your stomach, place your elbows under your shoulders so that you lean on your forearms. Take a few deep breaths and allow the muscles in the low back to completely relax. Stay for two to three minutes. Another first-aid exercise used mainly to treat severe low back pain, this should always follow Exercise 1 and be done once per session.

- **Exercise 3: Extension in Lying.** Lying on your stomach, place your hands under your shoulders. Slowly straighten your elbows and push the top half of your body up as far as you comfortably can while completely relaxing the pelvis, hips, and legs, and allowing your low back to sag. Hold for a second or two before lowering to starting position. With every attempt, try raising a little higher until your back is extended as much as possible with your arms as straight as possible. McKenzie calls this the most effective first-aid procedure for acute low back pain, also useful for treating stiffness and preventing pain's return. For treatment of pain or stiffness, repeat ten times per session, with sessions spread evenly six to eight times throughout the day.

- **Exercise 4: Extension in Standing.** Stand upright, with feet slightly apart, placing your hands on the small of your back with fingers angled toward the spine.

Bend backward from the waist as far as you comfortably can, hold for a second or two, and return to starting position. Each time, bend a little farther. During acute pain, this exercise may replace Exercise 3 if you cannot exercise in the lying position. After full recovery, this is McKenzie's main tool in preventing further low back problems. Use it whenever you will be working in a forward-bent position— *before* the pain starts.

• **Exercise 5: Flexion in Lying.** Lie on your back with legs together, knees bent, with your arms at your side. Bring both knees up to your chest, place your arms around them, and gently pull your knees as close to your chest as you can. After a second or two, lower to starting position. Do not raise your head during the exercise, or straighten your legs as you lower them. Each time, try to pull your knees a little closer. This exercise relieves low back stiffness; perform it carefully, only five or six times per session, with sessions three to four times per day. Follow this and all flexion exercises with a session of Exercise 3. You can stop doing this exercise when you can easily pull your knees to your chest without tightness or pain, at which time you can progress to Exercise 6.

• **Exercise 6: Flexion in Sitting.** Sit on the edge of a steady chair with your knees and feet well apart, and your hands resting between your legs. Bend forward and touch your hands to the floor. Return immediately to starting position. Each time, try to bend a little farther. The exercise can be intensified by holding your ankles and pulling yourself down. Do this only after you've completed one week of Exercise 5. In the beginning, do only five or six times per session, with sessions three to four times per day. Always follow with Exercise 3.

• **Exercise 7: Flexion in Standing.** Stand upright with your feet well apart and your arms hanging loosely by your side. Bend forward and run your fingers down your legs as far as you comfortably can, then immediately return to upright position. Each time, try bending a little farther. Do this only after you've completed two weeks of Exercise 6. At the start, do only five or six repetitions per session, with sessions once or twice per day. Always follow with Exercise 3. For three months from the time you have become pain free, Exercise 7 must *not* be performed in the first four hours of your day.

Source: Treat Your Own Back, by Robin McKenzie. With permission of the McKenzie Institute and Spinal Publications New Zealand Ltd.

SMART SOURCES

American Physical
  Therapy Association
1111 N. Fairfax St.
Alexandria, VA 22314
800-999-APTA
703-706-3248
www.apta.org

Canadian Physio-
  therapy Association
2345 Yonge St.,
  Suite 410
Toronto, Ontario
Canada M4P 2E5
800-387-8679
416-932-1888
www.physiotherapy.ca

Both these organiza-
tions provide infor-
mation about the role
of and referrals to
physical therapists.
APTA, the certifying
body for physical thera-
pists in the United
States, also sponsors
periodic toll-free
hotlines to answer
questions on the treat-
ment and prevention of
back pain and offers a
variety of free bro-
chures, including
"Taking Care of Your
Back."

rest was widely advocated, benefit from lengthy terms of bed rest, according to a recent study published in the *New England Journal of Medicine*.

With extended bed rest, muscles weaken, bone mass can decline, and disks can miss out on nutrients that are "pumped" into them by physical activity. "After a few days you begin losing ground instead of gaining," says physical therapist Bill Boissonnault. The drawbacks aren't all physical, either. The longer we stay in bed, the harder it can be emotionally to return to work, wean ourselves off medication, and summon the motivation to heal. Feelings of disability and depression can take hold.

Of course, this doesn't mean you should keep going and going until you're a goner. "We don't want the message to go out that no matter what, someone shouldn't have bed rest," says Dr. Kuritzky. Trauma victims need rest in order for their wounds to heal, and for some back pain sufferers, the anguish is so excruciating that lying down is the only option until the pain eases up. The point is that in most cases a day or two is usually enough; and, even then, getting up every few hours for a brief walk around the house is encouraged.

Do You Need a Physical Therapist?

"We love getting people in the office before the problem arises—when they're looking for an appropriate exercise program in advance of any pain," says Orthopaedic Section President Bill Boissonnault of the American Physical Therapy Association. "But pain is usually their motivating factor."

Many physical therapists (also called PTs, or physiotherapists) practice in hospitals, but more than 70 percent are in private physical therapy offices, health and rehabilitation centers, sports facilities, and other venues as well. In many if not most cases, your first contact with a physical therapist will stem from a doctor's referral. (In fact, in many states, that's the only route allowed; see below.) On occasion, current or recovering back pain sufferers who know the value of exercise—and its potential risks—initiate contact themselves prior to starting a fitness program.

"Not everybody who has pain needs to see a physical therapist," says Boissonnault. "When pain begins to interfere with someone's lifestyle—their social responsibilities, family responsibilities, their work—that's when it's time for intervention."

Like other back-care-oriented professionals, the PT will use the first visit to take your history, review any medical records provided by your doctor, and conduct a physical evaluation. "Usually by the time we get to see a patient, the majority of red flags [of serious back injury or disease for which surgery might be necessary] have already been cleared," says Kim Dunleavy, an orthopedic specialist who notes that the PT is thoroughly trained in what to watch for should a red flag have been overlooked, or should a new symptom appear. Of course, physical therapists can play an important role in postsurgical recuperation as well.

While a physician might focus on treatment and cure of the injury or disease, physical therapists focus on functional changes to ease the pain, prevent its return, and get you out and healthily going about on your own. What you want out of the treatment matters, too: Is it to compete in a marathon, or to be able to sit comfortably at your

SMART DEFINITION

Physical therapists (PTs) or Physiotherapists

Health care professionals who evaluate and treat people with health problems resulting from injury or disease. PTs assess joint motion, muscle strength and endurance, function of heart and lungs, and the patient's performance of activities required in daily living, among other responsibilities. Treatment includes therapeutic exercise, cardiovascular endurance training, and training in how to perform the activities of daily living. More than ninety thousand physical therapists practice in the United States today, treating nearly one million people every day. More than twelve thousand physiotherapists are licensed to practice in Canada.

Source: American Physical Therapy Association. Canadian statistics from the Canadian Physiotherapy Association.

What Matters

• Moving and positioning yourself in ways that pose minimal stress upon the back.

• Resting appropriately for the pain, then resuming normal activity as soon as you comfortably can.

• Maintaining a healthy level of physical activity and an appropriate amount and type of exercise.

• Getting qualified exercise guidance to prevent further injury

What Doesn't

• Extensive bed rest when you don't need it.

• "Olympic" level exercise or athletics programs.

• Doing it all "on your own."

office desk? "There are a lot of people who put up with the pain because they don't know that they can do without it," says Dunleavy.

After the evaluation, a treatment regimen can be tailored to your individual needs. Beyond the sort of individually tailored exercise program that, say, a personal trainer might design, a physical therapist also uses a great deal of passive manual therapy (meaning they do it to you)—moving or stretching a limb, applying resistance to strengthen a muscle group, manipulating joints, and other hands-on techniques to detect trouble spots, lead you in proper movement, and assess progress. Along the way, ongoing education is provided in proper body mechanics and posture as it applies to your particular lifestyle, weaknesses, and strengths.

Depending on your condition, your preferences, your physical therapist, and your insurance coverage, among other factors, you can opt to do your exercises home alone, in group classes at the therapist's office, in a hospital or outpatient facility, or a combination of these or other locales. Even if you're on the "shy" side, classes are often encouraged for their motivational power. "Patients get support just from being able to talk to others with the same conditions," says Dunleavy.

How to Choose a Physical Therapist

In the United States, physical therapists must have a four-year college degree in physical therapy, which can be followed by a master's degree in the field. After graduation, PTs must pass a state-

Sex Talk

Sex might not be the first thing on your mind when back pain has you down, but once the acute stage is over, your love life can resume. You'll even have the blessing of the American Physical Therapy Association: "The psychological and emotional benefits of a healthy sexual relationship may aid recovery," reports the brochure "Taking Care of Your Back," "and the pelvic motions of gentle intercourse are good exercise for conditioning your low back."

Just do take it easy at first; and try positions that pose a minimum of stress on your back and don't require you to bear too much weight—the "spoon" approach, with both partners on their sides, facing the same direction, is an example of one. For some, bending forward will cause pain, while for others bending back is the problem—there are no standard rules. In general, keep your knees bent; keep to slow and easy movements; if it hurts when you do something in one way, do something else; and do let your partner in on what you're going through.

"It is vital for you to keep in mind that you are not the only one having a problem with sex," writes physical therapist Lauren Hebert in *Sex and Back Pain*. "Your partner is also living with the problem. Direct open communication is the tool that will restore good sexual relations. . . . You can use new attitudes, better communications with your partner, and new approaches to enjoying sex to not only recover what you lost, but also to build a better sex life than you had before."

administered national exam to be licensed. Other requirements vary by state. So does your access to PTs: Currently, thirty-two states allow "direct access" to evaluation and treatment by a PT. Forty-six states allow direct access to evaluation only; for the rest, a doctor's referral is necessary.

Look for a licensed therapist who is an Orthopedic Certified Specialist (O.C.S.) who specializes in the back. The more advanced training they have, the better. Several types of advanced credentialing exist: certifications, clinical residencies, advanced master's programs. A therapist with the initials M.O.M.T. after her name, for instance, has a master's degree in orthopedic manual therapy.

Physical therapists can be board certified by the American Physical Therapy Association in a variety of specialties, from pediatric to geriatric. Certified specialists use the initials "C.S." preceded by the initial of their specialty area (as in O.C.S., above). Neurologic- and sports-certified PTs are appropriate for those with spinal cord injury or extensive athletic involvement, respectively.

• **Ask about credentials and education.** In addition to a state license, what other certification and degrees does he or she hold?

• **Ask about experience.** How many years have they been practicing? How much of that time has been devoted to treating the area of the back?

• **Ask about the practice.** What sort of patients do they see? What is the staff-to-patient ratio? Is there adequate assistance to allow enough time for you?

• **Take a tour of the facility.** Look not just at the PT's office but also at the area in which exercise programs are held. Be sure that the space is well-maintained and the equipment provides the variety you need. Also, is it convenient geographically and in terms of your schedule?

No matter how careful you are, there are times when back pain strikes and it doesn't seem as though it will ever go away. In the next chapter we explore the wide variety of approaches to help you feel better.

THE BOTTOM LINE

Although back pain can strike anyone, many of us can protect ourselves by replacing bad physical habits with better ones—and the sooner, the better. Even when you are already aching, the right movements and exercise under the guidance of a trained professional can help you heal.

CHAPTER 5

Relieving the Pain

THE KEYS

• As the body's warning system, pain should not be ignored.

• Used appropriately, over-the-counter and prescription drugs can safely block pain messages or reduce their effects.

• Mild electrical stimulation treatments can eradicate or ease pain.

• With or without the use of medications, an array of injection therapies provides pain relief.

• Pain centers offer hope for the millions suffering the physical and emotional torment of chronic backache.

Pain is the body's way of announcing that something's wrong—it's a healthy signal that can alert us to the immediate danger of touching a hot stove top or the threat posed by moving in a way that exacerbates a sprain. "Don't do it," our body is saying. "You'll make things worse." But chronic pain—lasting months or years—can pose threats of its own, affecting our daily lives and our emotional state and often generating depression, tension, and unhealthy "pain behaviors" that can cause more trouble—and more pain—still.

Happily, there is hope. A bewildering variety of pain relievers exists, from old-fashioned rest and relaxation; to high-tech spinal pump implants; to "deep brain stimulation," in which an electrode in the brain receives an electric pulse from a tiny generator implanted in the chest. Fortunately, most of us do not need the more extreme measures, but we can rest easier knowing they exist.

In the last chapter, we explored some of the more conservative pain-relieving approaches of stretches and exercise; here we look at the next steps, from over-the-counter painkillers to physician-administered methods of relief.

How Pain "Works"

Ever notice how you sometimes cut your finger and don't even know it until you see a blood drop, while at other times the slightest pinch can elicit a yelp? The amount of pain you experience depends not only on the injury but on your perception of it.

In simple terms, there are basically two types of nerve fibers: large nerve fibers, which carry messages having to do with sensations such as touch or pressure; and small nerve fibers, which carry pain messages. Both types of fibers are connected to tiny receptor cells in and beneath the skin, which send messages along the nerves, into the spinal cord, and up to the brain by an action called *firing.* Usually, the large fibers send more messages to be processed by the nervous system and perceived by the brain. When an injury occurs, however, the body produces chemicals at the site of injury that cause the small pain-transmitting nerve fibers to get more attention. Some of these chemicals, *bradykinin* and *prostaglandins,* cause the firing rate of the small fibers to increase; the prostaglandins also increase circulation to the area, causing swelling or inflammation (which, as we noted in chapter 3, is a way for the body to help heal itself). At the same time, *neurotransmitters* are produced within the nerve fibers which help transmit the pain message to the brain.

As the pain message is being sent, however, factors can come into play that affect how much of the pain you perceive. The sensation from the small pain fibers can be overridden or decreased, for instance, by increasing the messages coming from the large fibers. Massage and even low electrical current can help.

Another way to decrease pain is to block the incoming messages from the small fibers. One way to do this is to block the prostaglandins' effect by taking aspirin or other *antiprostaglandins.* Another class of drugs, *narcotics* or *opiates,* affects the perception of pain at the brain instead of at the site of injury.

The body itself also produces its own painkillers. Among them are endorphins, opiate-like chemicals found in the spinal cord and brain, which can be stimulated by exercise, laughter, relaxation, acupuncture, and other nonmedicinal means. (Even a placebo, a drug-free preparation given to those who believe they are receiving medication, can prompt the body's endorphin response.) Adenosine triphosphate (ATP), a chemical that allows us to tense our muscles, has also been linked with pain reduction.

Just as our emotions can lead to pain relief, our susceptibility to pain can be increased by our own fears, tensions, and even the duration of the pain itself. It has been shown that chronic pain increases the sensitivity of the small nerve fibers so that lesser degrees of injury can have greater effect.

All the more reason to catch pain as early as possible. "In some cases, symptoms and signs may be evident within a few weeks to a few months after the occurrence of an injury or the onset of disease," says the American Academy of Pain Medicine in "The Necessity for Early Evaluation of the Chronic Pain Patient." "The cause of pain is not always known or apparent. For many patients, initial medical evaluation and treatments effectively relieve pain that might otherwise become chronic."

Prescription and Over-the-Counter Medications

Prescription and over-the-counter medications to relieve pain tend to operate in one of several ways: at the source of the pain, where they slow the "pickup" of the sensation by the small nerve fibers, or at the brain, by slowing the perception of the sensation. Other medications work on the cause of the pain itself—reducing inflammation and easing muscle spasm, for instance—or help us along by allowing us to get some rest.

Like other methods of pain relief, drugs might not heal the source of the problem but they can be helpful adjuncts to rest, physical therapy, and other recuperative measures. They buy us time while the healing takes place. Most prescription drugs—especially strong, narcotic (opioid) medications that can lead to addiction—are recommended only for short-term help.

Analgesics

Available both over-the-counter and, in stronger doses, by prescription, these medications exist solely for the relief of pain. In the stronger, narcotic form, they work by depressing the central nervous system—slowing the brain's ability to perceive pain—but raise issues of dependence and tolerance, where more of the drug is needed to obtain the same effect. Safer, non-narcotic analgesics act at the site of the pain to reduce the stimulation of the nerve endings.

Nonsteroidal anti-inflammatory drugs (NSAIDs) relieve pain, stiffness, swelling, and other symptoms of inflammation in muscles and joints by blocking prostaglandins released at the site of injury. Among the most popular for back pain relief are ibuprofen (Advil, Motrin); naproxen (Naprosyn); and ketoprofen (Orudis, Oruvail).

Aspirin (acetylsalicylic acid or ASA) is an NSAID that deserves special mention. The best-known member of a family of drugs called *salicylates,* it traces its roots back to salicin, a substance in willow bark that helped ancient Greeks feel better as far

SMART DEFINITION

Pain physician

A specialist recognized by the American Medical Association, who focuses on the prevention, evaluation, diagnosis, treatment, and rehabilitation of painful disorders. The pain physician may serve as a consultant to other doctors or be the principal treating physician, providing direct treatment, prescribing medication and rehabilitative services, performing pain-relieving procedures, counseling patients and families, or directing a multidisciplinary team of health-care providers.

SMART DEFINITION

Centrally acting analgesics

Painkillers that affect the central nervous system.

Peripherally acting analgesics

Painkillers that work at the site of pain.

back as the fifth century B.C. (Another salicylate, Doan's Backache Pills, contains magnesium salicylate as its primary ingredient.) The world's most widely used drug, aspirin is consumed by Americans at a rate of 80 billion tablets a year, and the *Physicians' Desk Reference* lists more than fifty over-the-counter drugs in which aspirin is the principal active ingredient.

Some products combine aspirin with other ingredients: Anacin adds caffeine; Excedrin adds caffeine and acetaminophen (see below); Bufferin adds ingredients to reduce irritation to the stomach lining while the pill dissolves; Ecotrin is enteric-coated aspirin, which dissolves in the intestine rather than the stomach.

Acetaminophen (Tylenol), a "nonsalicylate analgesic," might prove easier on the stomach than aspirin and is comparable in painkilling effectiveness, but it doesn't relieve the stiffness or swelling of inflammation. Acetaminophen works by raising the pain threshold for temporary relief of minor aches and pains.

Narcotic analgesics, available only by prescription, act primarily on the central nervous system (and are called centrally acting analgesics), and change our perception of and emotional response to pain by binding with receptors there. Narcotic analgesics such as codeine and propoxyphene are most often used for the treatment of mild to moderate pain; while diamorphine, levorphanol, and morphine are used for the management of the most severe cases. Narcotic analgesics can be combined with the non-narcotic (peripherally acting) variety as well. The drugs Percodan and Percocet, for instance, are combinations of the narcotic analgesic oxycodone with the non-narcotic analgesics aspirin and acetaminophen, respectively.

Together, they can be more effective than either agent alone.

Muscle Relaxants

To reduce the pain from muscle spasm or tightness, muscle relaxants might be prescribed. Most work by slowing the signals from the brain that cause muscles to contract—and that means *all* your muscles, not just the ones causing the pain, so don't be surprised if after taking them your coordination is somewhat off. Methocarbamol (Robaxin), cyclobenzaprine (Flexeril), orphenadrine citrate (Norflex), and carisoprodol (Soma) are among those prescribed.

Tranquilizers

Antianxiety prescriptions can achieve the same effect as muscle relaxants at the same time as they relieve anxiety, which can be the exacerbator—if not the sole cause—of muscle tension. *Benzodiazapines,* among the central nervous system depressants, include alprazolam (Xanax), chlordiazepoxide (Librium), and diazepam (Valium), which is particularly noted for its use in relaxing muscles and relieving spasm.

Antidepressants

Very low doses of antidepressant medications— lower than would have an effect on psychological disorders—are sometimes prescribed to relax muscles, reduce pain, and aid the sleep of those with chronic backache. Among them are the *tricyclic antidepressants* clomipramine hydrochloride (Anafranil), imipramine hydrochloride (Tofranil), and amitriptyline hydrochloride (Elavil); and *SSR (se-*

F.Y.I.

Tranquilizers are often given to back-pain sufferers as a means of immediate relief from sometimes severe pain. User beware of these substances: while the short-term effect is relief from pain, the long-term effects of their use are dangerous and detrimental to your health and well-being. A serious side effect of their long-term use is tranquilizer dependence. And never should tranquilizers— or any other pain medication—be taken while consuming alcohol.

SMART DEFINITION

Steroids

A class of hormone, including estrogen, testosterone, and cortisone.

Corticosteroids

Synthetic reproductions of hormones secreted by the adrenal cortex. Glucocorticoids are corticosteroids that decrease inflammation and, in the process, can reduce intestinal absorption and increase excretion of calcium, among other things.

Anabolic steroids

Not the kind used to ease back pain. The term anabolic describes an ability to build tissue, such as muscle. Anabolic steroids, derivatives of the male hormone testosterone, increase metabolism and are sometimes abused by athletes in training to temporarily increase muscle size.

lective seratonin reuptake) inhibitors such as fluoxetine hydrochloride (Prozac), and paroxetine hydrochloride (Paxil). Less frequently used *monoamine oxidase (MAO) inhibitors,* such as phenelzine sulfate (Nardil), address "atypical" depression, which includes components of anxiety.

Other Anti-inflammatory Drugs

Corticosteroids are synthetic analogues of hormones secreted by the adrenal cortex. Prednisone is a glucocorticoid, a corticosteroid with anti-inflammatory properties. But there's a concern: They reduce intestinal absorption and increase the kidney's excretion of calcium.

Some medications combine several types of drugs. The powerful Parafon Forte C8, for example, combines the muscle relaxant effect of chlorzoxazone with the analgesics acetaminophen (non-narcotic), and codeine (narcotic) for relief of muscle spasm and pain associated with muscle injuries and cervical disk problems, among others. Chlorzoxazone, a centrally-acting agent, works primarily at the level of the spinal cord and brain, interrupting a mechanism involved in producing and maintaining muscle spasm. The combination of acetaminophen and codeine provides additional pain relief.

Taking Medication Safely

The National Council on Patient Education and Information calls it "the *other* drug problem." Every year, mistakes involving prescription and over-the-counter drugs can be linked to 125,000 deaths and up to $20 billion in hospitalization costs nationwide. Dangers range from prolonged illness and unpleasant side effects to endangered health. What you don't know can hurt you.

"The more you, the consumer, understand, the less chance there's going to be a problem," says Michael J. Smith, R.Ph., chairman of the New Hampshire Pharmacist Association, who stresses the importance of an open dialogue between patient, doctor, and pharmacist. "It's a matter of communication and rapport."

• **Know what you're taking.** Familiarity with the name and type of drug you are prescribed will help you detect pharmacy errors. Self-prescribed over-the-counter drugs pose risks as well. Read the label carefully and ask a pharmacist's advice.

• **Know where to store it.** Keep medication in its original container to remember what it is and how to take it. Use child-resistant caps if you have kids or pets; and don't keep drugs in a bathroom medicine cabinet, where humid conditions can affect the contents. Store in a dry place, away from extreme heat or cold.

• **Know what you're treating.** Some drugs are directed at relieving symptoms; others at a cure; still others at keeping a symptom-free condition, like high blood pressure, in check. The more you know about what the medication is supposed to do, the better you can gauge its effectiveness.

• **No more, no less.** Don't readjust the dosage on your own. If you feel a medication isn't working, or

F.Y.I.

Number of prescriptions written in 1998:
2.8 billion*

Percentage of Americans who currently use medications:
64 percent[†]

Percentage using prescription drugs:
49 percent[†]

Percentage using nonprescription drugs:
30 percent[†]

Source: National Council on Patient Education and Information, citing *National Association of Chain Drug Stores, and [†]*Parade* figures.

side effects are bothering you, call your doctor, who will alter either the dosage or the medication.

• **Know when to take it.** Before meals or on an empty stomach? On a round-the-clock dosage schedule or one based on waking hours? Learn what to do if you miss a dose: take it when you remember, double up next time, or just skip?

• **Know how long to take it.** Will you be taking the drug for a week or indefinitely? Until used up or on an as-needed basis? It is important for you to know how long a given drug will be part of your life, because certain drug-related lifestyle changes that are acceptable in the short term may be more difficult to maintain for long periods of time. If you are told to finish the dosage, do: even if symptoms seem to vanish, many conditions need continued treatment for a complete cure. Don't save any medication "for later"—drugs lose their potency over time. And never self-prescribe for yourself or others.

• **Know what to take it with . . . and what to avoid.** Other medications, alcohol, tobacco, caffeine—even certain foods, beverages, and vitamins—can dilute or magnify a drug's effectiveness, or cause hazardous side effects. Drug interactions and allergies are among the greatest dangers and the most easily avoided, thanks to computerized patient profiles and information sheets kept at many drug stores. Loyalty to one pharmacist with an up-to-date record will reduce risk, as will keeping a copy of your own records.

• **Know when to go generic.** Lower-priced generic drugs contain the same ingredients as brand name versions, but different manufacturing practices can affect their effect on you. Your pharmacist is not allowed to give you a generic brand without physician approval.

• **Know what activities to avoid.** Drug-related drowsiness or impaired judgment may diminish your ability to function safely, so heed those warnings about avoiding large machinery—including cars. Other drug-related changes in body chemistry can present dangers as well, such as medications that increase sun sensitivity.

• **Know the danger signs.** Some side effects are more worrisome than others. Ask your doctor or pharmacist which ones are cause for alarm.

• **Know the impact of medications on other aspects of your health.** People with diabetes, hypertension, or a history of heart disease or ulcer, and women who are nursing, pregnant, or planning to become pregnant are just some of those who should steer clear of certain drugs. Your doctor and pharmacist should be fully informed of your past as well as your present state of health.

The Truth Behind "Deep Heating Action": Liniments and Salves

Absorbine Jr., Mineral Ice, and Eucalyptamint are just some of the muscle rubs promising "temporary relief of minor muscular aches and pains resulting from overexertion and fatigue."

The most common ingredients in liniments—

methyl salicylate, menthol, and camphor—are known as *rubefacients* (Latin for "to make red") and work not so much by relieving the ache of your muscles but by taking your attention from it. They are, basically, irritants. Applied to the sore area, they cause blood vessels to dilate, which brings increased circulation and warmth (and redness) to the surface of the skin, along with some temporary pain relief. They are known as counterirritants: basically, you're distracted from your initial ache and pain.

Bengay's "penetrating pain relief" is due to methyl salicylate and menthol, with the "ultra-strength" formulation doubling the first ingredient and adding a little camphor for good measure.

Muscle rubs are available in alcohol-based liniments, which penetrate deeper into the skin, and in lotions, creams, and ointments, which stay on longer. Use only externally, on skin that is not broken, unusually sensitive, or already irritated. Stop if excessive skin irritation develops, and don't cover or tightly bind the treated area. To prevent severe burn, don't use a heating pad or other form of heat treatment (including hot showers or baths) in combination with a muscle rub.

Below are the most common ingredients used in liniments and salves.

Camphor

Used in natural or synthetic forms in many muscle rubs, ointments, lotions, liniments, and other pharmaceuticals as a weak antiseptic, a mild anesthetic, and a rubefacient.

Capsicum

A rubefacient, this is the resin in Cayenne pepper.

Menthol

A type of alcohol obtained from varieties of mint oils, this rubefacient has a mild anesthetic effect.

Methyl Salicylate (Oil of Wintergreen)

Probably the most widely used counterirritant, this may be produced synthetically from petroleum chemicals or naturally from the leaves of an evergreen shrub native to North America.

Phenol (Carbolic Acid)

Produced synthetically, phenol is used in concentrations of 1 to 5 percent as a preservative, disinfectant, and antiseptic. Found in a few patent medications, such as Campho-phenique and Phenolated Calamine Lotion, phenol has anesthetic and anti-itch properties.

Electrical Stimulation Therapies

As an alternative to pain-relieving drugs, a variety of therapies that use electrical impulses to block pain can be prescribed for patients to use on an as-needed basis. Most often used in conjunction with other pain-relief treatments, including physical therapy and exercise, electrical stimulation works either by "short-circuiting" or redirecting the pain message; increasing the body's ability to produce painkilling endorphins; or, in some cases, by relieving muscle spasm at its source, although exactly how they do this is not always known. Electrical

F.Y.I.

Muscle rubs, salves, and ointments to treat the temporary discomforts of back pain are available over the counter—that doesn't mean that they're always safe to use and will cause no side effects. These aids have powerful ingredients, and care must be taken when using these products. Always apply these only as directed, and never exceed the recommended amount to be used or the suggested duration for the product's use. Discontinue the use if you experience any of the side effects listed in the product's warnings.

stimulation is not recommended for those with a history of cardiac problems or for those who wear a pacemaker, and because the effects on fetuses are not known, it should be avoided during pregnancy. Treatment outcome may be affected by the use of drugs or the user's psychological state. Here are a few of the more common techniques.

Transcutaneous Electrical Nerve Stimulation (TENS)

Some say it works best for acute pain such as that associated with a pinched nerve; others say it's particularly well-suited to chronic pain; some say it works only as well as a placebo; others say it's among the best pain-easing options around. As inconclusive as the literature may be, one way or another, about 100,000 people use TENS each year for temporary pain relief.

TENS works by sending low-voltage electrical impulses from the surface of the skin to the nerve fibers just below, blocking pain messages from the nerves to the brain. It does this via small electrodes placed on the surface of your skin, usually in the area of the pain, and attached to a small stimulator—about the size of a small personal cassette player—that you wear and control, turning the TENS unit on and off as needed to control pain. The doctor who prescribes the unit will teach you where to place the electrodes and how to use the device, which can be rented or purchased. *Interferential current* is a similar approach.

Percutaneous Electrical Nerve Stimulation (PENS)

More invasive than TENS, PENS sends painless electrical impulses into muscles through fine needle electrodes. (It's been called electrical acupuncture.) A study published in the *Journal of the American Medical Association* involving sixty men and women with long-term lower back pain caused by degenerative disk disease compared PENS with TENS and exercise therapies. Each approach was used for thirty minutes three times a week for three weeks. PENS was found "significantly more effective" in decreasing pain after each treatment, as well as in improving physical activity, quality of sleep, and sense of well-being. Ninety-one percent of the patients reported it the most effective in decreasing their pain.

Spinal Cord Stimulation

Reserved for extreme cases of chronic pain, this method involves having electrodes implanted under the skin near the spine, connected to a small receiver located either below the collar bone or in the abdominal area. Activation of a stimulation transmitter that you wear cues the receiver to send low-current electrical impulses to the spinal cord, short-circuiting pain signals.

Injection Therapies

When nothing seems to help and pain is excruciating, a variety of injections may be used as a last resort before—or to postpone—surgery. After a physical exam and appropriate diagnostic tests have pinpointed the source, injections of local anesthetic (such as lidocaine or marcaine), corticosteroids (such as cortisone or Depo-Medrol), and/or other drugs into the tissue around the affected area or trigger points elsewhere in the body may be given to provide relief. The anesthetic blocks the pain's transmission to the brain and in some cases immobilizes the troublesome tissue; the steroid reduces swelling and inflammation. Some injections are given in the doctor's office, others in an outpatient surgical facility.

Injections usually provide a quick fix. However, for those with chronic pain or a history of problems, injections are only a temporary relief. "They're all ancillary to help with the pain," says Arnold J. Weil, M.D., of Rehabilitation Medicine Associates of Atlanta, a specialist in nonsurgical orthopedic medicine with a special interest in spine care. "The key is restrengthening and exercising the muscles and relearning proper body mechanics. These are just tools to help reach that goal."

Epidural Injections

To relieve inflammation, swelling, and pain that has a neurological source, this technique involves injecting a local anesthetic and/or an inflammation-reducing steroid into the epidural space, which is the space inside the spinal canal, between the outer membrane protecting the spinal cord and the ligament that supports it. Although the choice of drugs used depends on the area of the injection, in general, anesthetic is administered to quell pain, and steroids given to reduce the swelling of the disk and any surrounding inflammation that might be pressing on a nerve. Rarely, narcotics or tranquilizing agents might also be used.

The procedure takes anywhere from fifteen to thirty minutes, and can be performed either in the doctor's office or at an outpatient surgical facility. Although it can be done without the use of a fluoroscope (an X-ray that your doctor can view as he proceeds, akin to an X-ray TV), there are clear advantages to its use. "The fluoroscope maximizes your benefit from the procedure," says Dr. Weil. "One study showed that 30 percent of the epidural injections done by anesthesiologists are not even in the epidural space. Without a fluoroscope you can't tell."

Epidural injections take effect in two to seven days, and are often given in a series of three shots—depending on success—at intervals one week apart. You might feel soreness around the site of the injection for a day or two.

Although this popular technique has been used for years and has been credited with long-lasting relief of pain—sometimes for months or even years at a time—a study in the *New England Journal of Medicine* reported only short-term improvement in leg pain for sciatica patients receiving epidural steroid injections, and found the technique appeared neither to help patients avoid surgery nor to aid their recovery in the long run. Other studies report success rates of anywhere from 15 to 50 percent, with success dependent in many cases upon appropriateness of use.

Trigger-Point Injection Therapy

You might remember trigger points from the discussion of myofascial pain syndrome in chapter 3. Trigger point injection therapy is another popular, if somewhat controversial, injection option. Unlike epidural injections, the trigger point approach is used for musculoskeletal pain. Local anesthetic and/or steroid is injected into the fibers within a muscle to relieve muscle spasm, which has often resulted from soft tissue damage. Usually per-

SMART MOVE

Painkilling injections can work wonders for those in severe pain, but they're not the be-all and end-all we'd like. "The injection is the first phase," says Arnold Weil, M.D., of Atlanta. "I wouldn't just do an injection and say, 'Okay. We're done.' There's still strengthening and rehabilitation ahead."

formed in the doctor's office, it can take effect immediately or after as long as two days.

In *Back Talk: How to Diagnose and Cure Low Back Pain and Sciatica,* author Loren M. Fishman, M.D., mentions the use, in this type of injection therapy, of a medication called Botox (botulinum toxin type A), which comes from the same bacterium that causes botulism. Said to paralyze muscle in spasm and eradicate pain within ten to twenty days, the effects have been claimed to last for three to four months, often up to half a year. Dr. Fishman also notes that normal saline (sterile salt water) has been used in trigger-point injections to push apart compressed or constricted structures.

Other studies have found "dry needling" (injections without drugs) just as effective as those using anesthetic, or anesthetic and steroid, for some low back pain patients. One researcher theorized that achieving a local twitch response—an involuntary muscle movement—with the needle was the most important factor in success, an idea compatible with the intramuscular stimulation technique described on page 141.

Nerve Root Blocks

In chapter 2 we talked about diagnostic blocks, procedures during which radiopaque dye and a numbing anesthetic are injected in or around a structure (such as a nerve root, disk or facet joint) suspected of being amiss, to see whether the pain lessens when it is reached, and so confirm its source. Used to relieve pain, the same sort of procedure might be called a *therapeutic block.*

Less invasive than epidural injections, nerve root blocks involve the injection of anesthetic and/or steroid at the site of the nerve root where it emerges from the spinal canal. After a local anesthetic is administered, a fluoroscope helps the physician pinpoint the specific nerve root involved before the medication is injected. Usually performed at an outpatient surgical facility, the procedure takes thirty minutes to an hour.

Facet Joint Injections

Injections of anesthetic, steroid, or a combination of the two can relieve the mechanical type of back pain caused by strain, trauma, or structural problems in facet joints. As with nerve root blocks, a fluoroscope is used to properly guide the application of the drugs, in this case directly into or near the joint. And, as with epidural injections, a series of one to three injections at one-week intervals might be used, with the effect taking place within a week.

Intramuscular Stimulation

With this approach, which is often erroneously compared with acupuncture (see chapter 7), nothing is injected but the needle. Used to treat chronic muscle spasms and soft tissue pain often related to nerve root irritation, intramuscular stimulation involves the insertion of a needle or series of needles into trigger points in the muscle itself, which causes the muscle fibers to "twitch," breaking the tightness of the contraction, and allowing the muscle to relax.

A new technique called *automated twitch-obtaining intramuscular stimulation* (ATOIMS), developed at the University of Pennsylvania Medical Center in Philadelphia, uses a battery-powered gun to shoot fine Teflon pins directly into irritated nerve roots and spasmed muscle as swiftly as three times within two seconds. At the time of writing,

SMART MOVE

"The earlier people take their complaints to a knowledgeable source, and one that can look at them in a holistic fashion, the better off they're going to be," says Hubert Rosomoff, M.D., D.Med.Sc., of the University of Miami Comprehensive Pain and Rehabilitation Center. "The single-modality approach is not the way to go, particularly when you get to the chronic pain phase."

the ATOIMS device has received Food and Drug Administration approval for custom, clinical, and research use and is available only at the university.

The Pain Center Approach

By some estimates, more than a thousand pain clinics have opened nationwide in the past few years in response to the millions of Americans suffering from chronic pain. The best of the centers offer a multidisciplinary approach to deal with pain's many aspects—physical, emotional, and behavioral—and combine medical treatment, physical therapy, psychological counseling, and even detoxification programs for the many chronic pain sufferers who become dependent on narcotic drugs and other substances. Additional approaches might include relaxation techniques, biofeedback, hypnosis, and acupuncture, to name a few. Job simulation and work conditioning might be offered to help quell common fears about not being able to work or being reinjured on the job.

"A pain center is not a pain center is not a pain center," says Hubert L. Rosomoff, M.D., D.Med.Sc., medical director of the University of Miami Comprehensive Pain and Rehabilitation Center, at which, by Dr. Rosomoff's estimate, about 85 percent of patients are there for back-related pain. "You have to be very careful."

One major difference between the true pain center and the so-called pain clinic or pain management facility, according to Dr. Rosomoff, is the multidisciplinary approach. "We include not only

Gender Differences and Pain

When it comes to pain, the "fairer sex" may have cause to cry foul. Women report more pains overall, more severe and chronic pains, and pains in more body regions than men. "From childhood on," according to a report published in the *Journal of the American Medical Association*, "the way the sexes perceive, describe, and cope with pain often differs. Measures that alleviate pain in one sex, moreover, may not work as well or at all in the other."

Among some of the possible explanations: differences in our physical structure, in the way we perceive pain, and in the ways we deal with it, which is likely to be affected by cultural directives as well as social and occupational roles. Hormones play no small part, either. In a study of the effects of sex steroids on inflammatory pain, female rats were found to have lower pain thresholds than males—but that reversed when hormones from the opposite sex (estrogens for males, testosterone for females) were implanted.

The pain experienced due to disease is no exception. Men and women with cardiac disease, migraines, and cancer all showed pain differences, as did those with osteoarthritis, a common cause of back pain.

In a study led by Francis J. Keefe, Ph.D., professor of health psychology at Ohio University in Athens, daily pain diaries of men and women with osteoarthritis showed that women experienced 40 percent more pain and that they reported more severe pain. Women also were more likely to vent their emotions, seek emotional support, and view pain as a warning to slow down, or take other steps to deal with it—strategies that lightened the pain's emotional toll. The day after a pain-filled day, men were more apt than women to report negative moods. These studies imply, Keefe said, that men with pain would do well to emulate women's more expressive style of active coping.

disciplines in medicine but also those of industrial engineering and ergonomics, vocational counseling, psychology, psychiatry, physical therapy, occupational therapy, as well as neurosurgery, physical medicine and rehabilitation, pain medicine, et cetera—all the components of the various disci-

SMART SOURCES

American Chronic Pain
   Association
P.O. Box 850
Rocklin, CA 95677
916-632-0922
www.theacpa.org

"We seek to get members out of the patient role and back to being a person," says this nonprofit organization with chapters worldwide. A quarterly newsletter and other educational materials, self-help group activities, and other resources encourage those in chronic pain to take more responsibility for their own recovery and to lead fulfilling lives.

plines that may be required to treat the patient, all under one roof."

The success of in- or outpatient programs depends on the severity of the pain, the causes behind it, and the severity of the patient's reliance on narcotics or other substances. Psychological issues are a concern: "Anybody that's been in pain for a period of time is going to have behavioral repercussions—depression, anxiety—and that has to be treated simultaneously," says Dr. Rosomoff. "There are clearly psychological issues that pertain to all people in chronic pain. A pain center must be balanced in terms of its approach."

The time to consider a pain center is when your pain is chronic, is interfering with your life, and has not been helped by anything else. "Our patients don't come to us unless they've been around the horn several times. We see the most difficult patients, the ones other treatments have failed," says Dr. Rosomoff.

When a patient comes to the Miami center, for instance, he undergoes a multidisciplinary evaluation—a three-day process—by a team of specialists in different fields to determine his specific needs and design a program to meet them. Next is a conference including the patient, the evaluating team, and family members or significant others at which is discussed the areas of concern, what treatments are advisable, and what the likely outcome of treatment will be. In some cases, chronic pain might not be "cured" so much as be brought to a manageable level, allowing the patient to lead a satisfying, productive life.

As in other aspects of achieving back pain relief, participation in your own recovery is key to success at a pain center. Start out by taking part in choosing the right center for you:

- **Who is on staff?** Good pain centers take a multidisciplinary approach. What variety of specialists is on staff? How many are full time?

- **Who do they treat?** Do they make a distinction between acute and chronic pain? Do they specialize in a certain type of pain, such as back pain, or in a type of approach, such as holistic?

- **What is the aim?** Do they have a true rehabilitation approach that takes your daily life into account?

- **What are the facts?** Never mind the glossy brochures. Ask for hard data and outcome results of the facility's program as it relates to your specific problem. How well does the program actually work?

- **Who is the medical director?** "Many of the so-called pain centers tend to fit the character of the medical director," says Dr. Rosomoff. A center run by a psychiatrist may lean heavily on psychology and psychiatry, while one run by an anesthesiologist may place its emphasis elsewhere. But the philosophy as well as the specialty counts. Rosomoff, a neurosurgeon, came to the conclusion twenty-five years ago that many of those operated on for back problems might not have needed surgery at all, and he now concludes that "most if not 100 percent have soft tissue problems that benefit from stretching and mobilization rather than surgery."

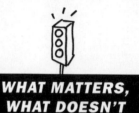

WHAT MATTERS, WHAT DOESN'T

What Matters
- Easing pain to a point that allows you to take rehabilitative steps and resume your life.

- Preventing long-term reliance on drugs.

- Acknowledging the psychological components of pain.

What Doesn't
- Temporary remedies that aren't complemented by other therapies for more-lasting relief.

- Pain treatment centers that promise one-technique "cures."

- The ability to ignore the pain. Problems need to be addressed if you're to live in good health.

No Quick Fix

As much as we wish we could promise it, no magic bullet exists to miraculously cure back pain. What pain-relieving medications and approaches can offer, however, is temporary relief, which breaks the pain cycle and allows a better opportunity for rest, physical therapy and exercise, and the curative powers of time to take effect. Used as a *supplement,* not as a replacement for other therapies, pain-easing techniques can seem like wonders indeed.

What works for one condition, of course, might not work for another. And short-term relief must be balanced with long-term effectiveness. Other issues to consider are accessibility and cost. One technique might be more effective in a research study, but another might be less invasive and more easily available for day-to-day use.

The elusiveness of back pain diagnosis also comes into play. An epidural injection might be of great help to someone whose problems stem from a herniated disk, but not for a person whose trouble has another source. Ultimately, the goal, of course, is not just to prevent or stop the pain, but to prevent or heal the cause. In chapter 6 we look at the ways in which surgery can—and cannot—help.

THE BOTTOM LINE

As useful as pain is as the body's alarm system, once we "get the message," most of us would rather it just went away and stopped interfering with our lives. Instead, it can seem to exacerbate the very problems of which it warns, and it may interfere with the steps we can take to get better. A wide range of pain-relieving medications and therapies can give us enough relief so that we can move on to the next step of recovery.

CHAPTER 6

Surgical Solutions

• For the small number of back pain sufferers for whom it is appropriate, surgery can bring welcome relief. The problem is deciding if you are one of those patients.

• By playing an active role in your own health-care decisions, you can increase your chance of successful recovery.

• Numerous approaches to back surgery involve everything from a walk-in visit to a local clinic to a few days in the hospital.

The good news is that the overwhelming majority of back pain sufferers don't need surgery to heal on their own, either completely or with only a small functional impairment to their daily lives. The bad news is that healing can take a fair amount of time, sometimes years. Severe, relentless pain has compelled hundreds of thousands of those with back problems to opt for surgical relief, propelling back surgery to among the most common types of operations performed. Here we take a look at what those operations are, and who needs them.

Do You Need Surgery?

When we think of elective surgery—that which is not life saving, but chosen—cosmetic procedures such as face lifts and tummy tucks are probably what spring to mind. The fact is, most back surgery falls into this category as well. Other than procedures performed for those with fractures or dislocations, infections, tumors, or other life-threatening diseases, many back operations are not absolutely necessary in the true medical sense of the word. Back pain alone—even if very severe—is technically not sufficient cause for surgery, nor is it something that surgery can necessarily cure. "Surgery has been found to be helpful only in one in one hundred cases of low back problems," according to the Agency for Health Care Policy and Research (AHCPR), which notes, "In some people, surgery can even cause more problems. This is especially true if your only symptoms are back pain."

If, on the other hand, your pain is caused by

neurologic rather than musculoskeletal trouble, or if you have any of the conditions mentioned above, surgery can help. An ongoing joint study begun four years ago by researchers from the Maine Medical Assessment Foundation, Massachusetts General Hospital, and the University of Washington at Seattle found that surgical approaches can offer better relief than nonsurgical treatment for patients with two common causes of low back and leg pain: sciatica, the lower back pain that radiates into a leg and is usually caused by a herniated disk pinching a nerve; and spinal stenosis, the narrowing of the spinal canal in the area of the spinal cord that can also compress nerves. In these cases, patients who had experienced symptoms for a shorter duration had better outcomes than patients whose symptoms had already been prolonged. Continued study has also revealed that in the stenosis groups, patients with symptoms in one leg fared better over time than those with bilateral symptoms. Long-term effects, however, won't be known for several more years.

The key is in having surgery for the right reasons, which is apparently not as obvious as it might sound. Appropriate patients, appropriate diagnoses, and the right approaches, performed correctly are key. Diskectomy—the operation to repair herniated disks—is one of the most common surgeries in the United States, yet population-based rates of this procedure vary widely around the country. Where the rates are higher—indicating, perhaps, less discrimination in who gets the operation and who doesn't—outcomes may not be as good.

Social, economic, and psychological factors also come into play. Just as they can significantly affect the response to back symptoms, they can have a big influence on the effectiveness of treatment

SMART SOURCES

AHCPR Publications Clearinghouse
P.O. Box 8547
Silver Spring, MD 20907
800-358-9295 or 301-495-3453

The "Patient Guide to Surgery and Pain" was developed by a private-sector, expert panel made up of doctors, nurses, other health care providers, an ethicist, and a consumer representative. The free booklet is available from the Agency for Health Care Policy and Research (AHCPR), an agency of the U.S. Public Health Service.
Call or write, and ask for publication number AHCPR 92-0068.

methods, including surgery. If a patient is depressed, lacks a social support group, or has financial problems, for instance, the success rate of any surgical procedure will fall.

With or without surgery, more than 80 percent of patients who have significant lumbar disk herniations will eventually recover, says Robert B. Keller, M.D., executive director of the Maine Medical Assessment Foundation in Manchester and coauthor of the above-mentioned studies. Though some people take longer than others.

Surgical Decisions

Michael and John have had the same symptoms, at the same intensity, for the same length of time. The same herniated lumbar disk shows up on their diagnostic tests, they are equally nonresponsive to all the treatment they have tried, and they have both heard the same list of risks and benefits for the same surgical procedure from the same physician. To operate or not? Michael says yes; John says no. Both can be right.

"If they are willing to be patient, they will both, in fact, probably get better," says orthopedic surgeon Robert Keller, who cites a Norwegian study that followed surgical and nonsurgical groups for six to ten years and found their outcomes to be the same. What's at issue, however, is the patient's willingness to wait. "You might say to yourself, 'He's telling me I'm going to be better in six years. Great,'" says Dr. Keller. "'Well, I don't know if I want to live this way for six years.'"

Shared decision-making is an important and well-recognized component of patient care. "Patients need to balance risks and benefits in their own personal setting," says Dr. Keller. "The physician is a very important player in the decision, but not the only one. The outcomes are better when the patient plays a role. Patients need to understand they do have choices."

Is the pain keeping you from going to work, or just from your weekly tennis game? Is your tennis game an integral part of your happiness, or just something you do to appease your spouse? Does the pain surpass your concerns about hospitalization, or does the fear of an inpatient stay at County General make the anguish easier to bear? No question or personal preference is too insignificant to count.

Just as your choice cannot be based upon the surgeon's word alone, neither should diagnostic tests alone be the deciding factor in whether or not you go ahead. Remember the study that revealed how many abnormalities appeared in the MRIs of people who didn't have any back pain at all. Again, a subjective measure carries weight.

"You don't need an operation if you don't hurt," says Steven R. Garfin, M.D., professor and chairman of the department of orthopedics at the University of California at San Diego, and past president of North American Spine Society. "Most people don't *need* an operation; they *choose* an operation because their quality of life is not adequate or comfortable. The surgery is for quality of life 99 percent of the time, and quality of life is a patient-directed choice. There's only one person who can make this decision—the patient."

STREET SMARTS

"All I wanted was for my doctor to give me a yes or no about surgery," recalls Brice, a fifty-one-year-old bank officer in Denver. "But she finally convinced me why it was important for me to make the choice. To do that meant I had to do a lot of learning, which I definitely wasn't up to, but really did help me know what I was doing and deal with recovery better than I probably ever would have otherwise."

When to Consider Surgery

Other than procedures performed for fractures, dislocations, tumors, or disease, surgery for back pain is most often an elective choice. Below are some of the situations that warrant serious consideration of invasive procedures.

• When your symptoms—leg pain, tingling, weakness or numbness, loss of bladder or bowel function—indicate a severe neurologic problem.

• After clinical evidence and diagnostic tests confirm your problem is one that a surgical procedure has been proven to help.

• When symptoms are severe to the point that they are disabling you or disrupting your life.

• When symptoms are persistent, and either don't improve or get worse.

• After you've given it time. Remember that most cases of back pain resolve themselves in six to twelve weeks. Decisions do not have to be made immediately; back surgery can usually wait weeks or even months without making the condition worse.

• When you've tried everything else.

Pre-Op Homework

From confidence in the ability of your surgeon to familiarity with the surgical options available to you, knowledge and preparation can go a long way toward reducing preoperative stress and increasing the chance of success, as well as bettering your ability to make the right decision about having the operation to begin with.

• **Examine your doctor.** Interview several surgeons, asking about their qualifications, how long they've been doing the procedure, how many they've performed, how many have been successful. Will you see the surgeon again afterward, or will you be referred to a physical therapist or other health care professional? Are you comfortable knowing this person will be operating on you?

• **Get a second opinion.** No reputable surgeon will take it personally. To the contrary, most will encourage you to seek another's view.

• **Put it in writing.** Things have a way of slipping our minds in doctors' offices. Write down your questions in advance, and bring a notepad to jot down answers. Here are just ten important questions you might ask:

1. What is the goal of this surgery?

2. How reliable are the diagnostic tests that support the decision for surgery?

3. What makes me a good candidate?

4. What is the success rate of this procedure on people like me?

5. How long has this procedure been offered? Is it experimental?

SMART MOVE

"You want somebody who specializes in spine surgery, whether an orthopedist or neurosurgeon doesn't really matter today," says Steven Garfin, M.D., of the University of California at San Diego, an orthopedic surgeon who trains neurosurgeons in spinal procedures. "Knowledge of the spine and knowledge of its mechanics are what matters."

6. How long does the procedure take? When can I leave the hospital?

7. What are the risks? What are the possible complications?

8. What are the benefits of the surgery?

9. How will I feel afterward? What sort of rehabilitation will I need? For how long?

10. How long will it take for me to get back to my usual life?

• **Share your history**. Discuss any surgical experiences you've had before and any concerns you may have, from anesthesia to scarring. Inform your doctor of any allergies, and tell her whether you are currently taking any medication (even birth control pills and vitamins).

• **Tie up the loose ends.** The smallest details of the briefest hospital stay can add stress you don't need. Prepare your travel route to and from the facility, and, if possible, enlist a supportive family member or friend (*not* a frazzled one!) to take you there and accompany you home. Pack a bag in advance, including a favorite photo, reading material, or whatever else makes you feel good. Arrange for home care if needed.

• **Practice relaxing.** Remember, tension makes back pain worse. Once you've made up your mind to go ahead with the surgery, put it out of your mind, and focus on your emotional health (see chapter 7).

Defining Success

The "success" of any approach to relieving back pain is far from an objective measure, yet success rates or outcomes carry a lot of weight when you're deciding whether to pursue that course or not. A procedure with a 90 percent success rate certainly sounds more promising than one at the 50 percent level. But—especially when it comes to invasive procedures such as surgery—the definition of "success rate" merits a second look.

"If your leg pain is gone, and your back pain is worse, you've had a successful operation," says one orthopedic surgeon, stressing that the only reasonable goal of most back surgery is relief of neurogenic pain such as sciatica, the symptoms of which are felt less severely in the back than in the limbs. Ask your surgeon about his or her goal. Make sure you know the answers to most of the following questions:

Does the success rate you're quoted refer to the total relief of back pain, or to an alleviation in its severity? Did it measure increased mobility, or improvement in strength? Were the results of a study gathered immediately after surgery, or a few years down the road? Are they generalized approximations, such as those in this book, or more narrowly focused statistics that apply to your situation? Were the subjects of the study people like you? In your age group? With your symptoms and diagnosis?

Were measurable, objective factors looked at, or were they the subjective opinions of those who've undergone the procedure? In the past five to ten years, improved research methods have used patient questionnaires that focus on outcomes relevant to them, not just relevant to their surgeons, with

SMART MOVE

When evaluating the type of surgery, focus on the probable outcome of the procedure, not the length of the incision involved. "If it's a four-inch incision and you have a ninety-plus percent success rate, it's better than a one-inch incision and a seventy percent success rate," says Steven Garfin, M.D., of the University of California at San Diego. "Ask how long you'll be in the hospital, how long it will take you to recover, not how long the incision will be."

queries related to such issues as whole body function, quality of life, expectations before surgery, and the telling question: "Would you do it again?"

Think about what "success" means to you. It might mean immediate results, or it might mean results that take longer to reach but are longer lasting. It might mean not the total eradication of pain but simply the ability to return to work, to pick up your grandchild, to take a long walk, or to garden for a few hours. On the other hand, faced with the prospect of surgery or hospitalization, you might "raise the bar" of your expectations. A 50 percent reduction in pain might be acceptable from physical therapy, for instance, but not from an invasive operation.

You can ask your doctor about surgery's potential dangers, but only once you've gauged your own definition of success can you really assess the risk-to-benefit ratio for you.

The Procedures

Although surgery isn't the answer to every type of back pain, sufferers of sciatica and spinal stenosis, among other maladies, can find it of help. Following, we describe the most common approaches for benign ailments, as well as some recent innovations.

Disk Surgery

One of the most frequently performed surgical procedures in the United States, diskectomy is by far the most common type of back surgery. Liter-

The Latest Is Not Always the Greatest

From tongue depressors to artificial hearts, from annuloplasty to diskectomy, every medical device and surgical procedure requires acceptance by the Food and Drug Administration to become approved for use in the United States. Although some criticize the FDA for foot dragging in comparison to the speed with which approvals are granted elsewhere in the world, others appreciate its rigorous pursuit of safety. Devices and procedures are not, however, held to the same level of intense scrutiny as the drugs reviewed by the agency. Also, if a procedure or device has previously been approved for use in another context and is considered to have undergone "evolutionary change," it can receive the FDA's nod for a new application with comparative ease.

Regard the latest innovations with a cautious eye. The new procedure you've just heard about on the nightly news might sound promising, but think twice before setting out for the medical center at which it's just been introduced. "People develop a lot of enthusiasm for new procedures and disseminate them broadly before adequate studies are done," says Robert Keller, who served on the AHCPR panel on Acute Lower Back Problems in Adults. "The public thinks, 'It's the latest technology and it has to be better,' but that's not always the case. We certainly don't want to inhibit new technologies, but they really need to be very carefully researched before they're released."

ally meaning "removal of the disk," the surgery may actually involve the removal of either all or, more often, a portion of a herniated disk to relieve pressure on or irritation of spinal nerves.

Diskectomy

For the standard, conventional diskectomy, a vertical incision about two inches in length is made along the midline of the back in the area of the troublesome disk. A portion of muscle is either cut through or moved aside to reveal the spine, and a small opening may be made in the lamina (the back part of the vertebra) to allow further access. (This procedure, called a *laminotomy,* should not be confused with a laminectomy, described later in this chapter.) Next, the nerve root is gently pulled back to reveal the herniation, and, with special instruments, most or all of the soft core (the nucleus pulposus) of the disk is removed to prevent the disk from herniating again. (The disk's tough outer casing—the annulus fibrosus—is usually left in place between the vertebrae, and, like the opening in the lamina, will fill with scar tissue within weeks.) Finally, the surgeon repositions the nerve and muscle, and the wound is closed. Success rates can be as high as 90 to 95 percent.

On average, diskectomies usually take about one hour, and are generally done on an inpatient basis, although outpatient procedures are not unheard of. Unlike years past, when patients might be confined to bed for lengthy periods, today most are up and walking within twenty-four hours and can be discharged from the hospital as early as the next day.

Microdiskectomy

Another "open procedure," microdiskectomy is similar to conventional diskectomy by most standards of measure. The difference: with the aid of visual magnification and instruments as small as two to three millimeters in width, surgeons can make a smaller incision, displace less muscle, and attain similar results, often on an outpatient basis. But don't let the size of the incision be your main focus, advises Dr. Steven Garfin. While an optical loupe may provide magnification at three and a half times that of the unaided eye, and a micro-scope seven to ten times, a certain amount of "elbow room," so to speak, will be needed by the surgeon once inside to do what needs to be done. That's what matters.

Percutaneous Diskectomy (Aspiration)

Among the newer and less commonly used meth-ods of disk surgery are percutaneous, or "through the skin" approaches. With this method, a part of the disk is sucked out, or aspirated, through a small opening via a narrow tube inserted into the disk's core or nucleus.

The benefits of percutaneous diskectomy, like other such minimally invasive surgeries, are that it can be done under local anesthetic in less than an hour, and patients can return to most normal ac-tivity within days. The less disturbance to the body's interior, after all, the less pain there is for the body to heal. But it is not for everyone: the pro-cedure can be up to 85 percent successful in cases where the outer disk material completely contains the nucleus. If not, pressure created during aspi-ration can force fragments of disk material out, causing other ills.

In its guidelines, the conservative Agency for Health Care Policy and Research (AHCPR) views percutaneous diskectomy with a wait-and-see ap-proach: "This and other new methods of lumbar disk surgery are not recommended until they can be proven efficacious in controlled trials."

Percutaneous Laser Diskectomy

This technique is similar to aspiration in its out-of-the-mainstream status, its minimally invasive ap-proach, and its limitations to cases in which disk

SMART DEFINITION

Minimally invasive surgery

Procedures character-ized by small incisions and the use of minia-turized instruments. The appeal: The less invasive a procedure, the less disturbance to the body, the less pain, the less scarring, the shorter the hospital stay, and the faster the recovery.

fragments have not strayed. After a fine needle is inserted into the nucleus of the disk, a tiny fiberoptic strand is sent through the needle. From this strand, bursts of laser energy can be directed to vaporize a small portion of disk material. The process causes pressure inside the nucleus to drop, and creates a vacuum that sucks the herniated portion of the disk back in, away from the nerve it is compressing.

The benefits of percutaneous laser diskectomy also resemble those of aspiration and other "through the skin" surgeries. On the downside: because the core of the disk is not removed, there is the possibility of recurrence, and long-term effectiveness remains questionable. If done appropriately, by someone adept in the technique, success rates have been estimated in the 65 to 70 percent range.

Endoscopic Diskectomy

A variety of microsurgical procedures can remove fragments of core material that have broken through the fibrous outer wall of the disk. For an endoscopic diskectomy, the surgeon steers a catheter equipped with a tiny camera lens (the endoscope) and minute instruments to cut and remove small disk fragments that are irritating a nerve.

Since the endoscope and the small tools can be guided through a small opening in the back, there is only minimal disturbance of tissue, and the hour-long procedure can be performed under minimal anesthesia on an outpatient basis. Still, studies remain to be published, and endoscopic diskectomy is not yet widely performed.

Intradiskal Electrothermal Annuloplasty

This new targeted thermal therapy, developed at the Stanford University School of Medicine in Menlo Park, California, uses heat to "seal" a herniating disk. During the outpatient procedure, a catheter equipped with a heatable coil is snaked through the disk under fluoroscopy. Then the coil is heated to a temperature approaching 200°F, which "tightens" the tissue, and seals the disk.

In Praise of the Papaya: Chemonucleolysis

Hailed with great enthusiasm when first introduced in the early 1980s, this rather controversial treatment—FDA-approved, then rejected, then approved again—involves the injection of the enzyme chymopapain to dissolve material in a herniated disk. The enzyme, which is derived from the papaya, has other purposes as well—just look at the ingredients on Morton's meat tenderizer.

The thirty-minute procedure, performed with the visual assistance of a fluoroscope, calls for a physician to inject chymopapain into the center of the disk while the patient is under local anesthetic. Proponents boast the absence of scarring, short recovery time, and a success rate as high as 75 percent when properly performed on the proper patient. Even the AHCPR calls chemonucleolysis "significantly" more effective than percutaneous diskectomy, if less so than standard or microdiskectomy. Nevertheless, although popular in Canada, Australia, and Europe, some poor outcomes and a few serious complications—quite possibly due to poorly performed procedures, or the treatment of inappropriate patients—have left it in relative disfavor in the United States.

"The experience of most of us who used it was it didn't work and most patients ended up back in the operating room having a standard disk operation and they were not happy," says Robert Keller. "People and physicians got disillusioned."

Before undergoing chemonucleolysis, patients should be tested for allergic sensitivity to chymopapain.

Treating one disk takes about one hour, and patients rest for thirty to forty minutes before going home. Two studies involving about sixty patients suffering from chronic low back pain of a diskogenic source reported "satisfactory" outcomes reaching nearly 75 percent. Patients required analgesics for one to three days afterward, and could return to work in one to five days. Post-procedure treatment included six weeks of self-guided, low-level exercise, followed by six weeks of physical therapy and rehabilitation. The better the catheter positioning, the better the outcome.

Long-term effects remain to be known and further studies are under way. "One of the questions people ask me—and I can't answer it yet, other than to give my assumptions and theoreticals—is what happens in two years, what happens in five years?" said procedure codeveloper Jeffrey A. Saal, M.D., clinical professor of functional restoration, in *Orthopedics Today*. "I think we will have some people that we can catch early on in their disk problem where they might have a small tear but an otherwise healthy disk. We can treat them and that might be the last we see of them. There are others who are on this cascade where the disk is going to degenerate and we'll need to treat them a number of times and keep them patched up—not perfect, but patched up to where they feel they are okay."

Laminectomy

Most laminectomies are performed to relieve neurogenic pain due to spinal stenosis—the narrowing of the spinal canal that can be caused by bony outgrowths, among other causes—and also to ease the pain of severe spondylolisthesis, a condition involving a crack in the vertebra. (See chapter 3 for more detailed descriptions of these and other conditions mentioned in this chapter.)

The process involves removing part or all of the lamina—the ridgelike back portion of the vertebrae that forms the arched "roof" of the spinal canal—to widen the spinal canal, clearing it of protuberances that may be compressing the nerves. In a total laminectomy, both the right and left portions of the lamina are removed; when only one side is removed, the procedure is called a *hemilaminectomy;* when performed upon more than one vertebra, the procedure is called a *multiple laminectomy.*

In time, scar tissue forms around the site, in a sense "replacing" the lamina and encasing the nerves. Depending on the type and extent of the procedure, patients can expect several weeks' recovery and physical therapy, and a success rate of 80 to 85 percent.

Spinal Fusion

Spinal fusion (also called spine stabilization or segmental stabilization) is performed to return stability to one or more segments of the spine that have become unstable due to such conditions as severe spondylolisthesis, fracture, injury, or even extreme wear and tear of the joints. Fusion might also be performed in combination with diskectomies or laminectomies in which the entire disk or a large amount of bone is removed.

During the procedure, slivers of bone about an inch long are removed from the patient's pelvic area (usually the sacral bone), and transferred to the unstable vertebrae, the surfaces of which are

F.Y.I.

In one year in the United States:

Disk removals or destructions:
273,000[*]

Spinal fusions:
160,000[*]

Laminectomies:
108,000[†]

[*] National Center for Health Statistics, National Hospital Discharge Survey, data for 1995 extracted and analyzed by the American Academy of Orthopedic Surgeons, Department of Research and Scientific Affairs.
[†] National Center for Health Statistics, National Hospital Discharge Survey, data for 1996.

roughened to prompt the body to start a repair process. There are two general types: *posterior fusion* and *interbody fusion*. With posterior fusion, the bone graft is placed on the back side of the vertebrae; with interbody fusion, the graft is placed between the vertebrae, where the disk has been removed. In both cases, the healing process causes the vertebrae to grow together, or fuse, creating a solid block of bone in the months following surgery, stabilizing and, in the process, stiffening the spine.

In some cases, surgeons can eliminate the need for the patient to have to recover in two areas of the body by using artificial bone or bone from cadavers instead of transferring slivers from the pelvis. In other cases, metal pedicle screws can be attached to the vertebrae at both ends of the area to be fused, affixing plates or rods to hold the area rigid while fusion takes place. Spinal fusions are usually done posteriorly, with the patient face down and the surgeon entering from the back. With the less frequent anterior approach, the patient lies on his or her back, and entry is from the front.

Drawbacks: Although it can claim a 70 percent success rate for treating back pain, fusions don't always completely heal (according to orthopedic surgeon Steven Garfin, the bones heal only 80 percent of the time). Complication rates of spinal fusion can be high, the procedure doesn't seem to make future surgery less likely, and there seems to be no firm scientific agreement on how to define spinal instability to begin with.

"We do more fusions in the United States than anywhere in the world, and the variation in population-based fusion frequencies is extraordinary," says Robert Keller, "which is a good indicator of uncertainty about whether it's appropriate. That always raises concerns."

"It's not a spectacular operation," says Dr. Garfin. "Most of the horror stories you hear about back surgery have to do with this. One should be very cautious."

Recovery

Once upon a time, back surgery patients stayed in bed—and in the hospital—for days, even weeks. But, just as it is for those suffering from an acute attack of pain, prolonged bed rest following surgery is a thing of the past. Within twenty-four hours, surgical patients are encouraged to sit up and, if possible, to stand and even take a short walk.

Under the supervision of a nurse or physical therapist, you'll be instructed in everything from the art of turning in bed to sitting up and getting to your feet to performing gentle exercise. You'll begin simply, with gentle stretches and flexes of the feet and ankles, working your way up to pelvic tilts and more.

Depending on your physician's availability, your condition, and, in many cases, your insurance coverage, you will either be scheduled with a physical therapist, and/or be given instructions for a gentle home exercise routine.

The length of time it will take you to be back on your feet can vary greatly, depending on everything from the type of surgery you've undergone, to the reason for it. Another variable is the lifestyle to which you'll be returning. A construction worker might need three months or so before being able to resume full-time activities, and even

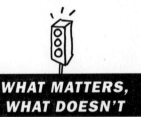

WHAT MATTERS, WHAT DOESN'T

What Matters

• That your condition is appropriate for the surgical approach.

• Recognizing that no surgical procedure can guarantee a permanent or complete "cure."

• Finding a surgeon who specializes in spine surgery.

• The outcome of the surgery.

What Doesn't

• Back pain alone, without suspicions of nerve root compression or other red flags, as a reason for surgery.

• The length of the incision.

• Success statistics that don't meet your criteria for success.

THE BOTTOM LINE

By far, most back pain sufferers will heal on their own within six weeks with conservative therapy—brief bed rest, pain medication, and a gentle exercise program—alone. Only about 5 percent will develop chronic pain that lasts longer than three months. Of those, surgery can prove miraculous for some, and useless for others. The challenge is to determine who is whom, which depends not only on accurate diagnosis, but on the patient's personal disposition and other unquantifiable factors. On the bright side: with appropriate symptoms and diagnostic tests, the likelihood of good outcome with surgery is high. Finding the right approach for the individual has a lot to do with its success.

then heavy lifting might be prohibited. Those whose days are filled with less strenuous tasks might be back in action within two to four weeks or less. Some activities, such as tennis, golf, or anything involving twisting, might need to wait a while longer.

Beyond the procedures mentioned in this chapter, other back surgeries offer hope—for example, rhizotomy, for those suffering the most extreme cases of nerve damage, which surgically severs a nerve to stop transmission of pain to the brain, or noninvasive proton beam radiosurgery, which uses the quantum wave properties of protons to remove spinal tumors. On the horizon are synthetic versions of disks, being used in other countries and just passing the experimental stage in the United States, which may offer another option.

But newer isn't always better. In chapter 7 we talk about some age-old approaches—and others—that are getting a new look.

Alterna-tive Answers to Relief

THE KEYS

• Off the traditional path, alternative approaches can provide a new world of relief.

• Whether the movement is passive or self-directed, body-work and movement therapies can "teach" our bodies how to heal.

• From the age-old practice of meditation to high-tech biofeed-back, mind-body medicine brings mental state and physical condition together.

It's often thought of as "New Age," but much of it has existed for thousands of years. "Alternative," "unconventional," "complementary," or "integrative" medicine—whatever you choose to call it—has been turned to for cures for everything from colds to cancer. And, for many, these off-the-beaten-path approaches are helping to relieve back pain.

What Is "Alternative" Medicine?

The use of the phrase "alternative medicine" describes a mixed bag of therapeutic approaches as diverse as chiropractic manipulation, creative imagery, and herbal remedies. The most widely accepted definition includes any treatment or health care practice not generally taught in medical schools, not generally used in hospitals, or not generally covered by medical insurance. But as more and more medical schools, hospitals, and insurance companies are including the formerly out-of-the-question practices, another definition may well be in order, and soon.

"There's a paradigm shift going on in American health care toward alternative medicine," says Jerome F. McAndrews, D.C., national spokesperson for the American Chiropractic Association (ACA), and on the advisory board of the American Association of Alternative Medicine, an organization dedicated to filling the void in communication between alternative health care systems and the public.

The eyes of the medical community were opened in January 1993, when Harvard physician

David Eisenberg, Ph.D., M.D., published a landmark survey in the *New England Journal of Medicine*. In 1990, the year of his study, Americans made 425 million visits to alternative care providers such as chiropractors, acupuncturists, and massage therapists—37 million *more* than the 388 million visits they made to primary care physicians. And in the great majority of instances, they paid out of their own pockets—roughly $10 billion's worth, according to the National Center for Complementary and Alternative Medicine (NCCAM). By 1997, the number of visits had risen to 630 million, and, reports a study in *American Medical News,* out-of-pocket expenditures rose to $27 billion.

Today, the National Institutes of Health (NIH) houses the National Center for Complementary and Alternative Medicine; three thousand conventionally trained American physicians have taken courses to incorporate acupuncture in their medical practices; at least 75 of the 125 medical schools in the United States offer elective courses in unconventional therapies or include these topics in required courses; and even the health insurance industry has begun to take note—and issue coverage—with NIH's blessings. Some managed-care organizations don't even require a primary care physician's permission.

Although all the methods described below can help relieve or prevent back pain, many of these less-conventional techniques fall into more than one "category" of approach. The Pilates Method, for instance, takes a mind-body approach to improving physical flexibility and strength. The yoga philosophy encompasses a lifestyle extending beyond how-to instructions for twisting yourself into pretzel shape. Some are more "alternative" than others: a massage therapist might be relatively easy

F.Y.I.

Complementary and alternative medicine encompasses twelve major health care systems, twenty-six "categories" of practice, more than 350 methods, and 10,000 ways of using them.

Source: National Center for Complementary and Alternative Medicine

SMART SOURCES

National Institutes of Health
National Center for Complementary and Alternative Medicine Clearinghouse
P.O. Box 8218
Silver Spring, MD 20907
888-644-6226
http://altmed.od.nih.gov

F.Y.I.

One of three Americans uses some sort of alternative medicine. Only 30 percent of them tell their doctor they do.

Source: Consumer Reports on Health

to find; a Feldenkrais practitioner might require a bit more searching.

Most important, there is a reason they are also called "complementary" medicine: they do not exclude, but can complement more traditional medical care. Reputable practitioners would not espouse an "I'm all you need" philosophy any more than a doctor would tell you not to go to a dentist. Remember: Seeing a chiropractor for back pain can be very helpful, but it doesn't mean you shouldn't know where the hospital emergency room is.

Bodywork

Used for diagnosis as well as healing, the laying on of hands is one of the most ancient types of health care. These touch therapies, therapeutic touch, or manual healing techniques—from acupuncture to zone therapy—are all based on a similar set of ideas:

• *Vis medicatrix naturae:* the philosophy that we can help the body to heal itself.

• Stimulating one part of the body can affect other areas as well.

• Blockages or misalignments of bodily structure (whether from the effects of gravity, injury, conditions at birth, or repetitive movement) throw the body off kilter. If we bring the body back into alignment, it will return to health.

Chiropractic

The relief of back pain has been synonymous with chiropractic from the very start. In 1895, Daniel David Palmer delivered the first chiropractic adjustment to Harvey Lillard, a janitor in his office with an aching back. From that one adjustment, Lillard, who had been deaf since childhood, would experience a full recovery—back, hearing, and all.

They won't claim to restore hearing to the deaf, but the 55,000 licensed practitioners of chiropractic today in the United States make it the third largest doctoral-level health profession after medicine and dentistry. Twenty-two million Americans turned to them last year alone for conservative management of back pain, neck pain, and headaches without surgery or drugs. "Natural, hands-on health care," in the American Chiropractic Association's (ACA) words. Ninety-three percent of the conditions that chiropractors see are musculoskeletal in nature; and back problems have been estimated to account for more visits than all other ailments combined.

Unlike massage, which deals with manipulation of soft tissue, chiropractic focuses on the relationship between skeletal structure (chiefly the spine) and function (the nervous system), finding and treating structural problems—from misaligned vertebrae to damaged joints—that can affect the nervous system. The doctor of chiropractic's (or D.C.'s) preferred prescription: annual checkups to *prevent* simple problems from affecting other parts of the system and worsening to the point of pain and dysfunction that are less easily remedied than those caught earlier on.

"If there's a loss of normal motion in one joint, for instance, the whole musculoskeletal system will

---

F.Y.I.

A statewide study led by researchers at the University of North Carolina in Chapel Hill found that of one hundred people who have back pain, about forty will see some type of health care professional. Of those who do, 39 percent will see a chiropractor first. Men were more likely to see chiropractors than are women, and younger people more likely than older back pain sufferers.

SMART DEFINITION

Spinal manipulation

Recognized by the U.S. Agency for Health Care Policy and Research as an effective therapy for acute low back pain, spinal manipulation is the traditional chiropractic tool to correct misalignments of the vertebrae, restore function, and reduce or eliminate pain. But while chiropractors are by far the largest group to employ the technique as part of back pain therapy, they are not the only ones. According to the American Osteopathic Association, 85 percent of doctors of osteopathy (D.O.s) surveyed use manipulative treatment in their practices. In smaller numbers, orthopedic surgeons and physical therapists practice spinal manipulation as well.

compensate for it," says the ACA's Jerome McAndrews, past president of Palmer College of Chiropractic (known in chiropractic circles as "The Fountainhead" for being the founding institution of chiropractic education) in Davenport, Iowa. "Medical doctors and osteopaths will look at where you hurt and treat it. The chiropractor will wonder if the pain site is the original problem, or if it's a sign of compensation from a problem elsewhere."

Chiropractic manipulation or adjustment is the most common treatment, where a doctor uses his or her hands to apply pressure or physical thrust to a joint. And no, you don't necessarily have to hear a "snap," "crack," or "pop" for the treatment to be effective. Gentle movements can sometimes do the job just as well. "The chiropractor had the image of a large, perspiring person twisting people in knots with loud crunching and cracking sounds coming from them," says McAndrews. Wrong.

Chiropractors may also use a variety of other manual, mechanical, and electrical therapies, including massage, heat and cold, electrical muscle stimulation, ultrasound stimulation of deep tissue, and other physiotherapy approaches, as well as wellness counseling in the areas of diet and exercise.

Although many medical insurance plans have yet to cover treatment from a D.C., the growing number of chiropractic enthusiasts might object to this being called an "alternative" form of care. Today, over 40 percent of auto and 35 percent of on-the-job injuries of all kinds are treated in the D.C.'s office; the Agency for Health Care Policy and Research recommends chiropractic spinal manipulation as the safest, drugless initial form of treatment for acute low back problems in adults; chiro practors now serve on over 250 hospital staffs; and the NIH is funding a Center for Chiropractic Research.

"The building of professional bridges is taking place at a rather dramatic pace," says McAndrews, who notes that over 50 percent of medical physicians now refer patients to chiropractors for low back pain. He, and many, are optimistic: "We're being called mainstream now."

Acupuncture

It wasn't until President Richard Nixon visited China in 1972 that most Americans would first hear about an exotic "needle therapy" called acupuncture, one of the most ancient forms of healing there is, dating back as far as 1000 B.C. The *New York Times* was hardly the first to report the approach. Centuries earlier, Jesuit missionaries returning from China coined the term acupuncture from the Latin *acus* ("needle") and *punctura* ("pricking").

Among the most thoroughly researched and documented alternative medical practices, and one of the most popular, acupuncture recently received the nod of a consensus panel convened by the National Institutes of Health, which concluded, "There is clear evidence that needle acupuncture treatment is effective" for a number of ills, from muscle pain to nausea. Panel members even spoke up for increased insurance coverage to allow more people "public access" to its benefits.

The technique has been used to treat osteoarthritis, headache, depression, stroke, and reduce dependencies on everything from drugs and alcohol to cigarettes and food. In the treatment of

SMART SOURCES

Chiropractic

American Chiropractic
    Association
1701 Clarendon Blvd.
Arlington, VA 22209
800-986-INFO
www.amerchiro.org

Acupuncture

American Academy of
    Medical Acupuncture
5820 Wilshire Blvd.,
    Suite 500
Los Angeles, CA
    90036
323-937-5514
www.medicalacupuncture.org

National Commission
    for the Certification
    of Acupuncturists
P.O. Box 97075
Washington, D.C.
    20090
202-232-1404

F.Y.I.

Conventionally trained U.S. physicians who have taken courses to incorporate acupuncture in their medical practices:
3,000*

Acupuncture practitioners in the United States:
6,500*

Number of patient visits per year for acupuncture treatments:
9–12 million†

Money spent on acupuncture by Americans per year:
$500 million†

* National Center for Complementary and Alternative Medicine.
† U.S. Food and Drug Administration.

back pain it has shown substantial therapeutic effect, with response rates cited from 50 to 80 percent.

The principle? Acupuncture is based on getting life energy—called *qi* (pronounced *chee*) and associated with electromagnetic charges that pass through *meridians,* or pathways, in the body—flowing right. Acupuncturists do this by gently inserting extremely fine needles at energy points that relate to vital organs and systems; acupressurists use pressure or massage; other related practices employ heat, friction, suction, impulses of electromagnetic energy, even laser. Six acupuncture styles are commonly used in the United States, including traditional Chinese medicine techniques, French energetics, and Korean hand acupuncture, each method with a slightly different orientation and approach.

Like electrical stimulation, and trigger point therapies (85 percent of trigger points coincide with acupuncture points), a direct effect of acupuncture causes spasmed muscle to return to its normal condition. In addition, acupuncture works in other ways, not all of which are understood. Many believe the process stimulates the production of endorphins, natural painkilling hormones and the anti-inflammatory hormone adrenalcorticotropin.

"If we look at muscular or neurogenic pain, I think acupuncture is ahead of almost everything else," says licensed acupuncturist Salvador Ceniceros, M.D., crediting its ability to reduce inflammation, "reprogram" muscles to their normal, prespasm state, and to stimulate specific neurotransmitters.

Dr. Ceniceros himself became interested in the technique in 1980 after bending over to pick up a box, throwing out his back, and having "tremendous problems" for over a year. Faced with the choice of ongoing medication or surgery, he took a friend's advice and tried what had formerly been a mere curiosity. After his third acupuncture treatment, his pain was almost completely gone, and he was enrolled in a three-year training course at UCLA.

Like other alternative approaches in this chapter, acupuncture has its limitations: when back pain is related to a structural disorder, such as spinal stenosis or osteoporosis, it can help relieve acute flare-ups but in the long run other approaches can be of greater help. "If the back pain is secondary to an arthritic change or facet syndrome where there are anatomical changes to the joints themselves," says Dr. Ceniceros, chief resident in the department of psychiatry at East Tennessee State University and the James H. Quillen V.A. Medical Center in Johnson City, "acupuncture can help reduce some of the inflammation, but it's not going to be able to change the anatomical changes that have taken place. It won't rebuild the joints."

"Probably 6 percent of the population have used acupuncture," says Dr. Ceniceros, "and of them, I'd say the great majority is for back pain. It's the most common thing most people think about acupuncture for."

Acupuncture needles vary in length from 1.25 to 15 centimeters; and most are so fine that three can fit inside one of the needles your doctor might use to immunize you against the flu. Usually stainless steel and disposable, they may have "handles" wrapped in copper wire, and they can be kept in place from only a few seconds to more than an hour—usually for twenty to thirty minutes—de-

SMART DEFINITION

Moxibustion

An acupuncture technique in which an herb is burned—either directly on the acupuncture point or to heat a needled point—to heighten the effect.

SMART SOURCES

Massage and Body Work

National Certification
  Board for Thera-
  peutic Massage and
  Body Work
8201 Greensboro Dr.,
  Suite 300
McLean, VA 22102
800-296-0664
703-610-9015
www.ncbtmb.com/

pending on the goal of the treatment. Although it can produce a sensation of soreness, numbness, or tingling, most patients don't feel a thing, often falling asleep during treatment. With the proper technique, say some Japanese practitioners, you should be able to put the needle into a sleeping dog and not wake it up.

Therapeutic Massage

Massage therapy, or therapeutic massage, is more than just a terrific way to relax. The rubbing, kneading, pressing, and stroking is no mere indulgence, but a very substantial boon to health that can both speed recovery from and reduce the likelihood of injury. Musculoskeletal, circulatory, and nervous systems all can benefit.

This laying on of hands relaxes tensed muscles, improves circulation, helps remove metabolic waste, stimulates the release of pain-relieving endorphins, and physically distracts us from the problems of our world, which can lead to the tensed muscles in the first place. Considering how much back pain is thought to be caused by muscle spasm, massage can be a very effective method of relief.

"Where it's especially beneficial is when the back attack primarily consists of muscle spasms," says Elliot Greene, M.A., NCTMB, past president of the American Massage Therapy Association. Muscle spasm is one of the most common primary sources of backache and a frequent accompaniment to other causes of the pain. Release the spasm and loosen the muscle, and you'll be granted more flexibility and movement, and that helps healing as well.

Another benefit that's often taken for granted is the soothing quality of nurturing touch. "Sometimes when people have back pain, they develop a lot of anxiety about any touch or movement around the area; they feel fragile," says Greene, whose practice is based in Silver Spring, Maryland. "Massage can help them through that."

An indirect factor comes into play, as well, when chronic tension patterns are relieved in areas other than the back itself. Massage of the hamstring muscles in the back of the thigh, for instance, can relieve tension that effects the postural positioning of the pelvis, which affects the health of the spine and lower back.

Of course, there are limits. "Where back pain is being caused by structural damage to the spine, obviously in that case massage is going to be more of an ancillary treatment," says Greene. "It will help with the symptoms, but it won't [be a] cure."

"One of the subtle benefits of massage," he adds, "is it helps to increase body awareness. People begin to be able to listen to their bodies better and that's really important to keeping your back healthy [and to] prevent injury."

The ABCs of Certification

Here's a primer to help you in your search for the appropriate professional.

Chiropractic

D.C.	Doctor of Chiropractic

Acupuncture

Dipl. Ac.	Diploma in Acupuncture (National Commission for the Certification of Acupuncturists)
D. Acu.	Doctor of Acupuncture (Occidental Institute Research Foundation)
L. Ac.	Licensed Acupuncturist
R. Ac.	Registered Acupuncturist

Massage Therapy

CMT	Certified Massage Therapist
LMT	Licensed Massage Therapist
CNMT	Certified Neuromuscular Therapist
LNMT	Licensed Neuromuscular Therapist

The Many Modes of Massage

Although all forms of massage involve manipulation of soft body tissues (usually with the hands, but sometimes with the forearms, elbows, and occassionally even the feet) with the aim of returning those tissues to a healthy, normal state, there are a plethora of methods. Some of the more common include neuromuscular massage, which relies on circulation-stimulating pressure to break the stress-tension-pain cycle; shiatsu, a Japanese acupressure technique using finger pressure on the body's meridian points to affect channels of energy flow; and Swedish massage, the most familiar, combining long, deep, kneading strokes with movement of the joints.

Like neuromuscular massage, trigger point and myotherapy are pain relief techniques to relieve muscle spasms and cramping. Seven to ten seconds of pressure are applied to areas where muscles have been damaged and blood flow is reduced, and then the muscles are gently stretched. A relatively new favorite, aromatherapy is more than just a good-smelling sensory experience; this infusion of herbal components into the massage oil is designed to offer a variety of effects, from relaxing to toxin-relieving to invigorating.

Reflexology and Zone Therapy

It might look like foot massage, but reflexology traces its roots to ancient Indian, Chinese, and Egyptian civilizations and, like acupressure and other bodywork techniques, is based on the idea that stimulating reflexes in one area of the body can affect corresponding body parts.

In 1913, American ear, nose, and throat physician William Fitzgerald introduced a version of reflexology to the West. With the body divided into ten zones, with the hands and feet the most accessible communication terminals, zone therapy took its first step. In the 1930s, therapist Eunice Ingham is credited with taking zone therapy to the feet.

Both reflexology and zone therapy operate on the same basic premise, similar to that of acupuncture and acupressure: following injury, stress, or illness, the body is in a state of "imbalance," and energy pathways are blocked. The hands of a trained practitioner can detect these problems, and, by applying gentle pressure, can release the blockages and restore the energy to its natural healthy flow.

Treatment sessions are often relaxing and pleasant enough to be confused with massage, and usually last about an hour. At times, however, fleeting discomfort, nausea, or even tearfulness might be experienced when the congestion or imbalance is released.

Structural Integration/Rolfing

"Invigorated," "better functioning," and "aligned," might describe the feeling of someone coming out of a structural integration session. Also known as "Rolfing," a trademarked nickname for Rolfing Structural Integration, named after its developer, Ida P. Rolf, Ph.D., the approach is based on soft-tissue manipulation and movement education.

"This is the gospel of Structural Integration," Rolf wrote. "When the body gets working appropriately, the force of gravity can flow through. Then, spontaneously, the body heals itself."

Rolf, a Ph.D. in biochemistry, viewed gravity as the strongest physical force with which the body has to deal, particularly the connective tissues, which physically support the body and all its pieces and parts. While a healthy connective tissue (or

SMART MOVE

Rather than focusing on the type of massage you think will be helpful, focus on finding a well-qualified massage therapist who is experienced in the field. "There are so many different kinds of massage, it would be difficult for the average consumer to understand them enough to make a choice," says Elliot Greene, M.A., NCTMB, former president of the American Massage Therapy Association. "In most cases, massage therapists learn several methods, and a good therapist will select those that work best based on the client's needs." More than thirty thousand massage therapists are certified through the National Certification Board for Therapeutic Massage and Body Work in McLean, Virginia.

SMART SOURCES

Structural Integration

Guild for Structural
 Integration
P.O. Box 1559
Boulder, CO 80306
800-447-0150
303-447-0122
www.rolfguild.org

Rolf Institute of Struc-
 tural Integration
205 Canyon Blvd.
Boulder, CO 80302
800-530-8875
303-449-5903
www.rolf.org

myofascial) system is flexible, elastic, and resilient, Rolf followers say, the effects of gravity, injury, or unbalanced movement cause the body to "shift," and that can ultimately lead to muscles that are chronically tense.

Rolf found that by manipulating the myofascial system, she could "organize the imbalances," and bring on healthy posture and structural change. The results are greater flexibility, a feeling of lightness and fluidity, better balance, increased breathing capacity, increased energy, and heightened self-confidence.

The Basic Ten Series, also known as "The Recipe," involves ten hour-long sessions, during which the client lies on a table while the practitioner applies pressure with hands, arms, and sometimes elbows, while keeping the relationship between tissue, respiration, nervous system responses, and organization in gravity in mind. The client's role: to "breathe into" the area being worked on, make small movements, and discuss with the trainer the patterns of movement and use of gravity involved.

Practitioners of the technique are trained and certified by the Rolf Institute of Structural Integration and/or the Guild for Structural Integration. Others, including Hellerworkers, practice a similar technique.

The Mind-Body Connection

That our mind and body are connected might seem too obvious to even have to point out. But the ways in which our minds and bodies interact are regrettably often overlooked by the traditional medical point of view.

If anything, it is the negative impact of mind on body that has received noteworthy attention. *Psychosomatic* or *psychophysiological illness*—a disorder of the body whose cause is rooted in the mind—is a more familiar concept than "psychosomatic healing," after all.

Earlier, we discussed some of the ways in which our emotions can make us more susceptible to back pain, both chronic and acute (see chapters 2 and 3). Numerous studies have associated anxiety with muscle ache and physical weakening, arthritis and bone loss, and even higher levels of fat deposits in the body, which tax the spine. When anxiety causes a backache, the ache itself can then make us more tense, which can lower our resistance, weaken our coping skills further, intensify the backache, and on and on. Stress from anything from an unhappy marriage to an unsatisfying career can heighten pain and prolong its duration, as well.

The good news is that what goes on in our minds can also *help* us. "The mind/body/spirit model emphasizes that thoughts and behaviors influence health and well-being," according to the Mind/Body Medical Institute and Mind/Body Clinic at Boston's Beth Israel Deaconess Medical Center. "The awareness that mind and body interact has important implications for the way we view illness and treat disease."

Relaxation techniques, hypnosis, biofeedback, meditation and prayer, and yoga are some of the approaches that can help.

STREET SMARTS

"When my back goes out, one of the most helpful things I do for myself is to repeat, over and over to myself, 'You're going to be all right. You're going to be fine,'" says Erik, who shovels "the annual mountain of snow" in Buffalo, New York. "Whether it relaxes the muscles or whatever it does, reducing the fear that the pain won't go away works better than a lot of medications I've tried."

The Emotional View

The specialty of *behavioral medicine,* also known as *mind-body medicine,* is based on a model of health and illness in which the mind, the body, and the spirit are all interrelated. Patients are assessed not just according to physical symptoms, or diagnostic tests, but also in terms of their psychosocial environment: stressors, habits, risk factors, social network, workplace considerations, hobbies, and more.

"The term mind/body/spirit is used to describe the many complicated interactions that take place among your thoughts, your body, your spiritual well-being (that is, a belief that one's life has meaning and purpose), and the outside world," according to the Mind/Body Medical Institute and Mind/Body Clinic, which operate on the belief that by taking such interactions into account—complementing primary medical care with smart lifestyle choices—we can maximize health benefits.

One of its most notable approaches, developed by Herbert Benson, M.D., founder and president of the institute and chief of the division of behavioral medicine at Harvard Medical School, is the "relaxation response," a term coined by Dr. Benson to describe a way to undo the stress response and counteract its harmful effects. The physician, researcher, and best-selling author, who believes we're nourished by meditation and prayer, emotional expression and support, reports benefits in everything from PMS to HIV.

Back when the dangers we faced came from lions and tigers, our minds helped protect our bodies by calling for a surge of adrenaline when we were threatened. Our hearts would beat faster, our blood pressure would rise, our breath would come hard and fast, and our muscles would tense, providing the burst of energy and strength we needed for escape. Today, when psychological stress is our greatest enemy, we still experience this "fight or flight," or stress response, which, if sustained, can lead to a long list of physical ills.

You may have experienced the relaxation response effortlessly as you were lying on a beach in the Caribbean, or basking in the warm glow from the fireplace after a day on the slopes. But there are ways to elicit the response even in the midst of stressful events. Deep breathing, meditation, physical stretches, mental imagery, and other techniques described elsewhere in this chapter all help.

Bringing art and fresh-cut flowers into your life, saying grace before meals, and taking "news fasts" are some of the life-enhancement strategies advocated by popular New Age health guru Andrew Weil, M.D. Soothing music, candlelight, and long baths have long been the "chicken soup" to mental duress. "Sometimes it may do the trick just to understand that the pain can depart once your brain stops sending the wrong messages to your back. Think about restructuring the patterns of thinking, feeling, and managing stress that lead your nervous system to spasm," he advises on the "Ask Dr. Weil" Web site, which also mentions yoga, stretches, posture, and diet as being of help.

John E. Sarno, M.D., professor of clinical rehabilitation medicine at the New York University School of Medicine and author of *Mind Over Back Pain,* goes a bit farther when it comes to the emotional roots of back pain. Dr. Sarno posits that stress, repressed anger, and other psychological factors are just about solely responsible for what he calls tension myositis syndrome, or TMS, which he believes is back pain's major cause.

SMART DEFINITION

Naturopath
Diagnoses, treats, and cares for patients using a system of practice that bases treatment of physiological functions and abnormal conditions on natural laws governing the human body. Utilizes physiological, psychological, and mechanical methods such as air, water, light, heat, food and herb therapy, psychotherapy, electrotherapy, physiotherapy, and excludes major surgery, therapeutic use of X-ray and radium, and use of drugs.

Source: U.S. Department of Labor

Mind Control: Hypnosis and Biofeedback

Used to treat everything from eating disorders to migraines, hypnosis has been praised as a pain-fighter in the *Journal of the American Medical Association*. In contrast to the zombielike trance we see in movie portrayals, it's a comfortable state of deep relaxation. And you don't have to lose consciousness for it to work or do anything against your own will. To the contrary, it will work only if the subject chooses to take part.

Self-hypnosis can even be undertaken during a back-strengthening exercise routine. Monotonous, repetitive movement has built-in potential for inducing a relaxing, trancelike state. (If you've ever been walking along on the treadmill and been surprised by the beep of your session timer after what seems like you just began, congratulations. You've been there.)

Biofeedback operates on the premise that by becoming aware of internal, involuntary bodily functions (from brain activity to muscle tension to pulse rate), we can bring them under our control and improve our health and ability to function in the process.

The technique has been used to treat a long list of conditions, including muscle spasms, muscle dysfunction caused by injury, chronic pain, movement disorders, headache, and many other afflictions of body and mind, from insomnia to hypertension. Even the military has used it to reduce stress among recruits; and health insurance companies are accepting biofeedback therapy as a treatment method for an increasing number of ills.

According to the Association for Applied Psychophysiology and Biofeedback in Wheat Ridge, Colorado, the term "biofeedback" was coined in the late 1960s to describe lab procedures developed in the 1940s that trained research subjects to alter brain activity, blood pressure, muscle tension, heart rate, and other internal activities of which we're normally not consciously aware. With a biofeedback monitor providing auditory or visual information about what's going on inside us, the theory holds, we can get a handle on physical reactions and processes formerly thought to be beyond our reach.

For instance, a monitor might sound a beeper or flash a light whenever the small muscles surrounding the cervical spine tense, a common cause of neck and shoulder pain as well as tension headaches. To relax the muscles—and avoid or reverse the pain—the patient would need to slow down the beeping, which sounds like putting the cart before the horse, but, nevertheless, has been proven to work. In the process, the biofeedback patient learns to associate sensations from the muscles with levels of tension and so learns how to relax them on demand. And no, you don't need to stay "hooked up" forever: after biofeedback treatment in study group populations, people were able to repeat their response with no sensors attached.

Meditation, Faith, and Prayer

Whether through deep breathing, creative visualization, the repetition of a mantra, or church services; whether accompanied by physical movement, or confined to the mind—meditation and prayer have, for untold ages, been bringing their adherents a sense of peace they didn't need science to verify.

SMART SOURCES

Biofeedback

Association for Applied
   Psychophysiology
   and Biofeedback
10200 W. 44th Ave.,
   Suite 304
Wheat Ridge, CO
   80033
800-477-8892
303-422-8436
www.aapb.org

Hypnosis

Milton H. Erickson
   Foundation
3606 N. 24th St.
Phoenix, AZ 85016
602-956-6196
www.erickson-
   foundation.org

F.Y.I.

The number of American medical schools offering courses on spiritual issues has risen from three to more than forty in the past three years.

Source: Consumer Reports on Health, July 1998

Researchers today believe the medical impact of meditation might be traced to its effects on cortisol, a hormone released by the body in response to stress. Although cortisol is helpful during occasional "fight or flight" situations, its continual release in response to the daily stresses of modern life can inhibit the immune system and slow tissue repair. Meditation may slow or reverse this process. Studies of people taught transcendental meditation showed that they had cortisol levels 15 percent lower than before they had become meditators; another study found that long-term meditators had a drop in cortisol levels of nearly 25 percent.

Religious belief and faith are prompting "amens" from the scientific community. At the 1997 meeting of the American Association for the Advancement of Science, a review of 212 studies found three out of four showing evidence of the positive influence of religious belief on health. One theory: like meditation, prayer and ritual may slow the production of harmful stress hormones in the body. Studies have shown this kind of stress reduction can reduce muscle tension, chronic pain, and high blood pressure, among other things.

A Duke University study of the elderly found that those who attended weekly church services were 50 percent less likely than nonattenders to have high levels of the protein interleukin-6, associated with illnesses including osteoporosis. But church attendance isn't a requirement. The meaning, purpose, and greater self-satisfaction found in the lives of the spiritual are acknowledged as contributors to the effect.

"Studies conducted over the past ten years do seem to show that patients whose spirituality is an essential part of their lives recover faster than those without a belief system," reported a feature story in *American Medical News,* a publication of the American Medical Association.

Then there are other possibilities: A San Francisco General Hospital study randomly divided almost four hundred seriously ill heart patients into two groups. Half were prayed for, half were not, and none knew which group they were in. The prayer recipients had less need of antibiotics, suffered fewer health complications, and had fewer cardiac arrests.

"The evidence is forcing medicine to deal with the fact that faith makes a statistically significant difference in health and healing," says David Stevens, M.D., executive director of the Christian Medical and Dental Society, whose seminars train physicians to integrate faith with physical care. "To offer our patients a complete program of care, every doctor must learn to incorporate these faith factors that have been proven to promote healing and health."

Bert E. Tagert, M.D., an orthopedic surgeon specializing in sports medicine in Bristol, Tennessee, has not personally witnessed any X-rays returning to normal or other "easily documentable miraculous physical healing," but does credit faith with an improvement in symptoms among the patients with whom, and for whom, he has prayed.

"Is it because of the change in their attitude and their hearts that they improved, or was there a physical change in their body? I can't answer that," says Dr. Tagert, who does believe that anatomical changes can occur as the direct result of prayer. "Such a wide number of things cause back pain, and it is certainly one of the disorders in which one's emotional response and other factors going on in a person's life can drastically affect the perceived symptoms."

Following is just one way you can reap the benefits of meditation.

1. Once or twice a day, set aside ten to twenty minutes of private time to practice the "relaxation response" or get in touch with your spiritual side.

2. Get comfortable and eliminate potential disturbances during your private time. Don't let a ringing phone distract you.

3. Close your eyes, or focus on a pleasing image.

4. Try repeating a single word, phrase, or sound—for instance, "peace," "the Lord is my shepherd," or a gentle hum—to help focus your mind away from daily cares.

5. Relax your muscles, and breathe slowly and naturally, repeating your chosen word or phrase as you exhale.

6. Don't stress out about relaxing. If your thoughts wander or body tenses, just continue as best you can.

Yoga

Probably not the first thing to spring to the minds of those suffering from back pain, yoga can actually be a very good approach to improving flexibility and the ability to relax both mind and body. And you don't have to twist yourself into knots to do it.

More than a set of physical positions and breathing techniques, yoga is a meditative approach and a way of life that promotes more limber physical *and* mental states. Along with improved flexibility and muscle tone, yoga can offer the stress-reducing, bodily-function controlling, disease-risk lowering benefits of other mind-body techniques.

From the Sanskrit root *yuj* or *yui,* meaning to yoke, or unite, yoga in the true sense combines a belief system, diet, and exercise to integrate spirit, body, and mind. But you don't have to be a total convert to reap benefits. Studies have found that when large muscle groups repeatedly contract and relax, as in yoga-type activities, the brain is signaled to release specific neurotransmitters that prompt feelings of relaxation and mental acuity. Many stress-reduction techniques are based on its principles.

You don't have to be a contortionist, either (just ask the more than 6 million Americans who practice some form of the ancient art). Beginner-level classes and different yoga styles can accommodate every body's level. There are several popular types of *hatha yoga,* the sort that's related to physical exercise (as opposed to the at times sexually oriented *tantra yoga,* which you probably won't find offered in classes at the local gym). *Mantra yoga* uses the repetition of a word or phrase to focus the mind. *Pranayama yoga* emphasizes breath control. *Ashtanga,* also known as "*power yoga,*" involves energetic transition from one posture to another. The style known as *Iyengar* concentrates on precise body alignment and position. *Gentle yoga* and *flow yoga* are a few Americanized versions.

SMART SOURCES

Yoga

American Yoga Association
P.O. Box 19986
Sarasota, FL 34276
941-927-4977
http://users.aol.com/
amyogaassn

This not-for-profit, educational organization and yoga school offers free guidelines on how to choose a qualified teacher, and ideas on where to start looking for one, along with other general interest information about yoga. Send a self-addressed envelope with 55 cents postage.

Take a Deep Breath

The expression "as natural as breathing" may not serve us as well as it sounds. The fact is, the way most of us tend to breathe naturally doesn't provide the oxygen we need during times of stress.

When you're tense, you breathe from the chest, using more muscles and more energy to draw shallower breaths than you do when you practice *diaphragmatic* or *deep breathing*—breathing from "the gut," with muscles below the lungs.

Diaphragmatic breathing slows and calms you in many ways. It can lower your heart rate and blood pressure, relax muscles, and clear your mind. Not only will deep breathing supply the body with more oxygen but it will do so with less effort. It's one of the easiest, quickest relaxation techniques there is.

• Get physically comfortable, uncross your arms and legs, close your eyes.

• Clear your mind of distracting thoughts or images.

• Put a hand on your stomach and take a deep breath—feel your diaphragm expand—and hold it for two seconds. Then slowly exhale. Take another deep breath, and again hold it for two seconds. Again, slowly exhale, keeping your mind clear of distracting thoughts.

• Repeat until you feel relaxed.

Movement Therapies

Like touch therapies, movement therapies are based on the idea that our bodies start out healthy, or with relatively minimal imbalances, and then, whether by the way we move or sit or carry things or the way we live in general, we throw the proverbial monkey wrench into the works. While touch therapies right this wrong by palpating, pushing, rubbing, pressing, or otherwise maneuvering our tissue, muscle, or bones, movement therapies teach us how to move and use our bodies in ways that can correct the harm.

With some approaches, you can do the movement; with others, a practitioner moves you to teach you how; others use a combination of both.

Pilates, or "The Method"

Don't let The Reformer, a wooden apparatus with cables, pulleys, springs, and sliding boards frighten you away. The Pilates (pronounced *puh-LAH-teez*) Method that uses it offers a mind-body approach to fitness that focuses on improving flexibility and strength, bettering the ways in which we move, heightening body awareness, and improving function along the way. "It's not just exercise," as Pilates practitioners would say.

Usually conducted in small group classes, the series of controlled movements performed on specifically designed equipment has gained great favor among numerous recovering back pain sufferers. Developed by Joseph H. Pilates seventy years ago, the practice boasts Martha Graham and George Balanchine among the first of many dancers to use it; today Hollywood celebrities have popularized the nonimpact technique. The focus is on the abdominal and back muscles—referred to as the body's core—in a routine of very few, but extremely precise repetitions of movement, and breathing patterns that don't always follow the exhale-on-exertion pattern of traditional exercise.

"People shouldn't have the kind of back pain that people have," says Joan Breibart, president of the Physicalmind Institute in Santa Fe, which

SMART SOURCES

Pilates and Similar Techniques

Pilates, Inc.
890 Broadway, 6th
   Floor
New York, NY 10003
800-4-PILATES
www.pilates-studio.com

Physicalmind Institute
1807 Second St.,
   Suite 15
Santa Fe, NM 87505
800-505-1990
www.the-method.com

teaches Joseph Pilates's approach. Breibart stresses that it's the ways in which we live and move that exacerbate physical imbalances we're born with and cause a great deal of the pain. Weak abdominal muscles and stiff backs, she says, are one result. "We end up with a very bad imbalance between strength and flexibility [or the lack of it] that stops us from moving in the way in which the body was intended to move. With the correct understanding and awareness, and exercises that strengthen the abdominals and improve flexibility of the back muscles, this is a problem that can be solved."

Trademark issues have some studios calling their Pilates-like technique "The Method," the Physicalmind Workout, or even "The P Word." Floor-work classes and home-use videos are available as well.

The Alexander Technique

Shakespearean orator Frederick Matthias Alexander summoned his greatest applause not on the stage, but with the technique he developed after he got a case of chronic laryngitis and traced muscular tension as the cause.

Neither a treatment nor an exercise, the Alexander Technique has been called a re-education of body and mind. Based on a concept called "primary control," which focuses on the relationship between head and neck, it encourages a return to the body's natural poise and coordination, where processes work efficiently as an integrated, dynamic whole. The "student" plays an active role in learning how to do this by gradually acquiring the skills it takes to correct the lifetime of nasty habits that cause physical and emotional stress.

Most often taught on an individual basis during thirty- to sixty-minute lessons, the technique is conveyed via "hands-on" work. A teacher observes the student's posture and movement patterns, and places her hands on the neck, shoulders, and back to learn about the student's patterns of breathing and moving, and what he may need to do differently. Twenty to thirty sessions are suggested, with a minimum of ten.

After one class, says one teacher, "a very typical reaction is the experience of lightness in movement; of lightness in themselves."

The Feldenkrais Method

"Exercise alone isn't enough," writes Lawrence W. Goldfarb, Ph.D., of Mind In Motion, in Santa Cruz, California. "Most of us are unaware of how we move. We pay attention to where we are going or what we are doing, not to how we move."

The Feldenkrais (rhymes with "ice") Method teaches us how to become aware of how the body works. "It helps your awareness so that you can perform at a higher level," says Debbie Ashton, M.S., a Knoxville-based practitioner who worked with the Olympic kayakers in the 1996 Games and has helped horseback riders and ski instructors, as well as "civilians" of all stripes.

Its developer, Moshe Feldenkrais, D.Sc., was a Russian-born physicist, judo expert, mechanical engineer, and educator. He was familiar with psychology and neurophysiology and a patentee of a number of sonar devices on the side. After crippling knee injuries, Feldenkrais taught himself to walk again.

The Feldenkrais Method was born and, with it, a way to improve posture, balance, and breathing;

SMART SOURCES

Alexander Technique

North American Society
 of Teachers of the
 Alexander Technique
3010 Hennepin Ave. S.,
 Suite 10
Minneapolis, MN
 55408
800-473-0620
www.prairienet.org/ale
 xandertech/nastat1.
 html

Feldenkrais Method

Feldenkrais Guild of
 North America
524 Ellsworth St. S.W.
P.O. Box 489
Albany, OR 97321
800-775-2118
541-926-0981
www.feldenkrais.com

WHAT MATTERS, WHAT DOESN'T

What Matters

• Not doing harm in the pursuit of healing. In other words, get a proper diagnosis first, to make sure you're not overlooking a serious medical condition that calls for a less conservative method of care.

• A properly trained and certified practitioner.

• The appropriateness of the therapy for your particular condition.

• Telling your doctor about any other treatments you are using, including self-prescribed health-store remedies.

What Doesn't

• Limiting your boundaries to conventional approaches.

• Using one method to the exclusion of others.

• What works for friends.

enhance coordination and flexibility; and gain some new patterns of thinking, to name a few benefits. "The thing that's different is you learn to do things for yourself that are specific to you," says Ashton. "If you can prevent bad habits from accumulating, there's less wear and tear on your whole system."

Taught in group "Awareness Through Movement" classes, during which a teacher verbally leads a sequence of moves; or through individual "Functional Integration" lessons, in which the teacher guides your movements with his or her hands, Feldenkrais relies on gentle movement and directed attention to get its message across.

"Feldenkrais is gentle," writes Goldfarb. "The idea is that you will change most easily if the new movements are more comfortable than the old ones. I like to say that our motto is 'No pain, *more* gain.'"

Weighing the Alternatives

Off-the-beaten-path approaches can offer new and possibly better answers to relieving back pain. On the other hand, we tend to know a lot less about them, and what they can both do to and for us. Tread carefully on new ground. Here are some useful guidelines that will help you explore the possibilities.

• **Be sure it's appropriate for you.** Some approaches are better for some things than others—yoga, for instance, may be great for flexibility, but it's a bad idea if you have any cardiac concerns. Decide what you want to get out of the experience, and find out if your expectations are in line.

• **Check references.** Talk with people who have been massaged, who have meditated, who have sat in "lotus position," or whatever you plan to do—preferably finding students of the practitioner you plan to be using. Scientific trials can provide solid clinical evidence of an approach's effects, but a personal view provides information you can't get from cold, hard stats.

• **Examine the practitioner.** If it's not conventional treatment, conventional rules and regulations are not going to be in place. Be sure the practitioner is licensed or regulated according to the laws of your state. Ask how long he's been in practice, what schools he's attended, what professional organizations he's a member of, what certifications he holds. A conventional variety of wide-ranging questions are your best bet.

• **Contact a national organization.** National groups familiar with state licensing, certification, and registration laws can often provide referrals and information about specific practitioners. Local and state health regulatory agencies and consumer affairs departments can also be helpful, and will inform you of any other clients' complaints.

• **Check out the office.** It won't tell you how effective or safe the treatment is, but it can matter when you're choosing who's practicing on you. Visit. Ask how many clients are typically seen in a day or week, and how much time the practitioner spends with each.

STREET SMARTS

"If my massage therapist hadn't asked whether I felt any tingling down my leg, I never would have known to get to my doctor, and who knows how bad off I'd be," recalls Chris, a thirty-three-year-old bartender in Chicago. Whatever form of relief you seek, be sure to tell the practitioner—in detail—about the type of pain you're feeling, and its source. When does it occur? How long have you had it? Have you seen a doctor? Sharing information can help greatly in the success of the treatment or, in some cases, direct you to a more appropriate source of help.

• **Consider the cost.** Many alternative treatments are not reimbursable by health insurance, but increasing numbers are. Regulatory agencies and professional associations are good resources for finding out what you might expect to pay.

• **Tell your doctor.** To prevent harm and aid success, both conventional and alternative practitioners should have a complete picture of what you are doing.

In the next chapter, we turn from techniques to technology, as we review the plethora of back-pain-relief gadgets and products of all kinds on the market today.

THE BOTTOM LINE

Alternative approaches to back pain relief are gaining attention—and acceptance—even amidst the conventional health care community. Among other signs that less traditional approaches are here to stay: 85 percent of insurance programs today provide coverage for chiropractic; and the number of physicians prescribing therapeutic massage is on the rise. More doctors and patients alike are realizing that more than one approach can help.

Available on the Market

From contraptions that suspend us upside down to automatic Chinese ear acupuncture devices to grape seed and pine bark extracts, a seemingly endless number of products are now on the market to relieve back pain. Some $2.5 billion was spent on such products, reported *Time* magazine, in 1995 alone. And business continues to boom.

Along with the more traditional items such as heating pads and high-quality mattresses, specialized back-relief emporiums springing up throughout North America are stocking water-filled pillows, "magic finger" neck massagers, cushions that vibrate in response to the sounds of the TV . . . It is not possible to list all the ergonomic innovations, the gadgets and the gizmos, much less review them all here. Instead, this overview of some of the more popular items will give you a view of the market, along with some consumer advice.

The Classics

As dazzled as we may be by all the high-tech innovations that promise back pain relief, some of the approaches mother taught us still work best.

Cold

Cryotherapy, the use of cold, is the time-honored, unchallenged remedy for reducing swelling, increasing circulation, and limiting inflammation. If you're looking for something fancier than a plastic bag to fill with crushed ice, a variety of cold packs can be purchased, including reusable gel packs that can be cooled in the lower part of the refrigerator before use, and items like the Chillow Cooling Pillow Insert, which can be slipped between pillow and pillowcase and reclined against for cushioned relief.

The sooner you apply cold, the better the results, and the general recommendation is to do so during the acute stage of pain, within the first twenty-four to forty-eight hours (see chapter 2 for acute and chronic pain dos and don'ts). To avoid potential harm to skin and tissues, avoid direct contact between the frozen substance and the skin. Wrap the pack in a towel or some other buffer, and don't apply for more than twenty minutes at a time. Let your skin temperature return to normal before another session.

Heat

If cold treatment is first aid, heat is second. *Thermotherapy* can help relieve muscle pain and soreness and hasten recovery when used after the first forty-eight hours of discomfort.

Heating pads, hot water bottles, clay or gel packs, or liquid sodium acetate containers—some microwaveable—are some of the many delivery systems available to increase circulation and decrease muscle spasm. Another option: heat lamps that employ soothing infrared light to temporarily relieve aches and pains. (Be careful not to confuse with sunlamps, which are often sold next to heat lamps in stores.)

To avoid burns, do not use any heat source on areas that are insensitive or where circulation is severely restricted; while you are sleeping; or if you are diabetic—you might not feel the damage.

STREET SMARTS

"I've seen a lot of high-tech, 'designer' ice packs for sale lately, but Green Giant frozen peas have always served me just fine," says Autumn, a graphics artist in St. Louis.

SMART SOURCES

The Virtual Corset, a lightweight box the size of a pager that's held against the chest bone with a few light straps, issues a warning vibration whenever the wearer slouches or bends—postures linked with a great deal of back pain. "It's kind of like having your mom around," says Steven W. Arms, president of MicroStrain, which manufactures the device. "We're not claiming to help people's back pain, just to help them stand or sit up straight."

The device, currently being used in a clinical and research capacity, is available to the public from MicroStrain for a hefty $795. A less-expensive version for consumer use is pending additional study.

MicroStrain, Inc.
294 N. Winooski Ave.
Burlington, VT 05401
800-449-3878
www.microstrain.com

Their use also should be avoided near areas where you've had surgery. To prevent burning yourself, test the devices before touching them to your skin. And never combine thermotherapy with topical liniments or salves (see chapter 5).

Braces and Corsets

Nonprescription back braces and corsets can provide helpful support and prevent back strain by keeping the wearer from bending at the waist. Neck collars, too, can restrict movement and relieve pressure on sensitive nerves during recovery from an acute attack of pain. Similar, supportive belts are recommended to pregnant women who are suffering from sacroiliac pain.

But whether the solid brace or the flexible corset, use these devices sparingly: long-term use can actually lead to dependency and, if worn long enough, to weaker, atrophied back muscles.

"I like back braces very much for one to two hours," says Tyler Cymet, D.O., of Sinai Hospital of Baltimore, who notes that our joint memory does not last longer than that. "They provide support and a reminder [of good posture], but only if you put them on immediately before an activity such as lifting. In the long run, corsets and braces can be more harmful than helpful. They do provide some joint stability, but they're not a long-term panacea."

Newer Arrivals

As helpful as it is to apply new knowledge to the use of old standards, time and progress have added some worthwhile options to the arsenal of back pain relievers from which to choose. Be a smart consumer. Some new "miracle" devices on retailers' shelves call for a healthy dose of old-fashioned skepticism, and some may provide their greatest benefit by lightening the heft of your wallet.

Supports, Cushions, and Rolls

Lumbar supports are lightweight, elastic belts worn around the lower back to provide support and prevent injury, and they can be helpful—if you wear them. According to an article in the *Journal of the American Medical Association,* researchers at Vrije Universiteit in Amsterdam studied 312 cargo workers of an airline company in the Netherlands to assess the impact of lumbar supports and education about lifting. After six months, compliance with wearing the support was found to be low (43 percent) and not significantly effective in reducing the incidence of low back pain or sick leave among the intervention groups. But in a subgroup of workers who reported having low back pain at the start of the study, use of the supports reduced the number of days of pain from 6.5 to 1.2 days per month. Like other forms of bracing, remember, the support is most useful when the device is worn for a maximum of one to two hours, and it can actually be harmful over a long period of time.

Lumbar support is also the term used to refer to cushioning devices such as lumbar rolls that bolster your lower back while you sit. Available in models appropriate for office chairs, car seats, even for reading in bed, the right model will fit the curvature of your spine and be thick enough to provide adequate support without pushing you too

F.Y.I.

Four major chains—the Healthy Back Store, Better Back Store, Relax the Back, and JoAnne's Bed & Back Shops—reported combined sales of $75 million in one year. Since then, the Better Back Store has been purchased by the Healthy Back Store.

Source: U.S. News & World Report

far forward in the seat. Many are available in a choice of shapes, sizes, and densities, and can be secured to your furnishings—or yourself.

Massagers

From folk-art-style wooden rollers that resemble children's playthings to computerized, motorized "built-ins," the number and variety of devices available to vibrate, pummel, and otherwise massage sore muscles is staggering. Some attach to the palm or back of the hand; others can be held by long, curved, reach-the-far-spots handles; and still others can be placed against a seatback or be laid flat on a bed, or are built in to a chair or mattress. Some have heating elements; others offer an array of speeds or stroke patterns. And they range in price from a few dollars to the thousands.

All work on the same principal as that of massage itself (see chapter 7), although mechanical massagers cannot claim the expertise (or overall effectiveness) of a certified therapist. The advantages: there's no need for an appointment, and they can indeed help your muscles to relax, stimulate circulation, and make you feel better. Used with liniments and muscle rubs (remember, no liniments should be combined with the use of heat), massagers can increase the penetration of the analgesics as well.

On the lower-tech end of the scale, the Jacknobber, a device resembling an overgrown children's toy, can be used to give a massage over light clothing, or with massage oil. Some massagers are "more aggressive" than others. A hefty device appropriately called the Thumper Pro, which is actually on permanent display in the Hockey Hall of Fame, provides deep tissue massage different from the rubbing, orbital action most devices use. Invented by a chiropractor, it uses a patented tapotement stroke, a pulsating, pounding type of motion (the manufacturer compares it with acupressure) promised to stimulate and energize tired muscles or, at least, distract you from your initial back pain. The lighter Thumper Mini-Pro personal self-massager offers heat and three power settings to adjust to thicker or thinner muscles.

Inversion Devices

Feeling batlike? A product such as Hang Ups will let you suspend yourself upside down. No bat cave needed. A less jarring alternative: inversion tables that let you start out upright and invert as much as you want as the table slowly tips back. In a word: self-traction. The theory: the upside-down posture allows the vertebrae to separate, relieving pressure on disks and providing temporary relief from back pain.

"You get the sense that you're literally growing a few inches," says Cliff Levin, executive vice president of the Healthy Back Store, one of the largest nationwide back-store chains, who's been known to invert himself before starting his workday. "You get a real sense of relaxation and well-being."

"Gravity inversion works wonders on back pain," said Milton Fried, M.D., of the Milton Fried Medical Clinic in Atlanta, in *The Doctors Book of Home Remedies*. "Gradually doing inversion traction with a proper, safe inversion apparatus for five or ten minutes a day will really work to rid you from lower back pain."

Others take a more cautious view when asked if devices like gravity boots are a good idea. "I don't

SMART SOURCES

Backworks
800-361-7788
www.backworks.com
Based in Winnipeg, Manitoba; catalog available.

The Healthy Back Store
800-4-MY-BACK
www.healthyback.com
Twenty-four stores throughout the United States; catalog available.

JoAnne's Bed & Back Shops
800-SOS-BACK
www.backfriendly.com
Sixteen stores in the mid-Atlantic and northeast United States; online catalog.

Relax the Back Store
800-290-BACK
www.relaxtheback.com
Over one hundred stores throughout the United States and Canada; catalog available.

think they're out-and-out dangerous, or are doing harm," says osteopath Tyler Cymet, who notes that they won't be of help if the problem is muscular pain. "Usually they're good if people have mild disk compression, which is the only time when traction can help. So if you use them and experience even more pain," says Dr. Cymet, "you've got your diagnosis."

Those with a potential for glaucoma should not use this approach; for all others, doctor's approval is a good idea.

Magnets

In wristbands and insoles; pillow inserts and mattress pads; seat cushions and self-adhesive disks; elbow, knee, and ankle wraps; even clothing and jewelry, magnets are attracting a following of fans who believe they can relieve muscle or joint pain and heal injuries. Used by healers in ancient Greece, China, and Egypt, magnet therapy has been touted as a cure for everything from insomnia to impotence and depression, and the devices are popular sellers in athletic, back, and mainstream department stores, by mail order, and via the Internet.

How do they work? There's no shortage of theories. Some believe magnets stimulate blood flow to the affected area (perhaps by acting on the iron in blood cells), bringing extra oxygen and nutrients while reducing toxins. Others hold that the magnets affect the way pain signals are sent along the nervous system, or that they otherwise interact with the body's electrical processes.

Anecdotal success stories abound, especially among athletes, reports the *Seattle Times*: "*Golf Digest* magazine reports that about eighty pros on the

PGA golf tour use magnet therapy to alleviate muscle aches, back pain, and arthritis. *Skiing* magazine reports that Olympic gold medalist Tommy Moe has used small magnets on his injured knees; top senior golfer Jim Colbert tapes magnets to his back before he plays; and Steve Atwater of the Denver Broncos sleeps on a magnetic mattress pad."

But no major studies have shown any pain relief effect, and scientific evidence is scant. According to Stephen Barrett, M.D., founder of Quackwatch, a nonprofit corporation dedicated to combating health-related fraud, although pulsed electromagnetic fields have been demonstrated effective for treating slow-healing fractures and shown promise for a few other conditions, few studies have been published about the effect on pain of the small, static magnets marketed to consumers.

Baylor College of Medicine did find an effect among fifty patients with diagnosed postpolio syndrome and muscular or arthritic-like pain. After wearing magnetic devices on painful points for forty-five minutes, 76 percent of the patients reported a reduction in pain, compared with 19 percent whose magnets were fake. On the other hand, a New York College of Podiatric Medicine study found magnetic insoles worn for a four-week period by thirty-four patients with heel pain didn't perform any better than nonmagnetic insoles. An ongoing University of Virginia study funded by the National Institutes of Health is researching the effects of magnetized sleep pads on patients with fibromyalgia, the painful muscle and soft tissue condition described in chapter 3.

One of the arguments against the therapy cites magnetic resonance imaging (MRI), which exposes patients to fields hundreds of times stronger

SMART SOURCES

We don't usually recommend commercial Web sites for information on the products they sell, but the easily navigated MotherNature's Encyclopedia of Natural Health, researched and written by health care professionals from a variety of disciplines, gives an honest assessment of what works—and what doesn't—along with cautions and caveats. Find the site at:

www.mothernature. com/ency

than those of therapeutic magnets but hasn't been known to heal any injuries.

"What's good about magnet therapy?" says Tyler Cymet, "It keeps people in business. People are making a lot of money from it, but, as far as the back, I don't see it increasing circulation or doing what it claims to do."

Although in most cases, magnet therapy won't do any harm, pregnant women and people with pacemakers or other electronic implants should avoid them.

Unlikely Back Aids

What is a document holder doing in a back store? Why are they selling inserts for shoes? Not all back aids are applied directly to or, indeed, come anywhere near our spinal columns, but *can* they help?

Office Aids

Whether you work at home or at corporate headquarters, a wide range of options is available to better the officeworker's back. Document holders that either prop papers up on the desk or that can be attached to the computer monitor can keep work at the proper level to avoid neck strain and unnecessary twisting. Attachable arm supports are now available that can be added to almost any desk or workstation. Some models of adjustable footrests can even encourage a rocking motion to stimulate circulation.

Entire office systems are available to conform to the ergonomic recommendations we shared in chapter 4. Some are geared especially for computer users, many are height-adjustable. For other tasks, or for workers on the move, there are alternatives such as the portable Ergo Desk available at Relax the Back stores, which has an inclined work surface and a folding second platform for reading materials. And the only problem with the incredible array of available seating options is that they might almost tempt you not to get up at all.

Accessories can help, too. Desk jockeys will find that taking a work break to flex the hands with exercise putty or grip balls, or even to roll around on an exercise ball to loosen tight muscles, can help relieve tension in the spine and elsewhere. (Though a stretching break and walk around the office every twenty to thirty minutes is a better idea.)

Herbals and Supplements

In addition to the alternative therapies discussed in chapter 7, a number of herbal remedies for back pain can be found on the market. You might find herbs bearing such colorful names as horsetail *(equisetum arvense)*, which, when mature, produces stems resembling a feathery tail and is said to have connective tissue–strengthening and antiarthritic abilities. Or devil's claw *(harpogophytum procumbens)*, a native plant of southern Africa, named for its shape and prized for its anti-inflammatory and analgesic properties.

Creams containing capsaicin, a pungent chemical derived from cayenne peppers, can relieve muscle or joint pain. Creating a burning sensation, especially the first few times it's used, capsaicin works by stimulating the nerves to exhaust their supply of a neurotransmitter needed for pain signals to be sent. Boswellia, a traditional Indian herbal remedy, is credited with relieving pain and stiffness, improving joint function, and having an anti-inflammatory effect.

Among the more popular "miracle remedies" are glucosamine and chondroitin sulfates, thought to help the body repair damaged or eroded cartilage. "Used right, for two to three months consistently, glucosamine sulfate can help," says Dr. Cymet of the substance, which occurs naturally in the joints. He cautions that chondroitin sulfate, however, like other supplements on the market, won't really help relieve joint pain unless injected. If ingested? "You won't get worse, but it won't cure anything."

The same can be said for the amino acid DL-phenylalanine (DLPA), boron, hydrolyzed cartilage, and many other supplements on the market. At best, they might help, or will simply relieve you of your money with no physical harm to you. At worst, however, they can hurt. Do not take these or any medications if you are pregnant, being treated for a medical condition, or are taking other drugs. For safety's sake, it's wise to check with a health care professional, trained nutritionist, or naturopath to be sure.

Shoes and "Wearables"

Just because they aren't worn on your back doesn't mean shoes and other "wearables" don't have a major impact upon its health. Not only do our feet serve as the body's shock absorbers, but they have a major effect on the ways in which we walk and stand. And if they're not happy, chances are our backs won't be, either.

Shoes have a lot to do with that happiness—and we're not just talking about the aesthetic joy of owning a pair of Manolo Blahniks. Feet that are inclined at unnatural angles from high heels, squeezed into pointy-toed pumps, aching from painful bunions, or pounded on noncushioned insoles will strain muscles and tendons, alter the distribution of body weight, and misalign the way we walk, throwing the rest of the body out of alignment, and stressing the spine. A wide array of insoles—from cushy foam styles to gels—and orthotics are available on the market to provide cushioning and support.

Other items can affect gait and posture as well. Overstuffed shoulder bags, even the heft of our wallets, can throw us off kilter given enough time.

Smart Advice with Wearables

• **Change shoes regularly.** Don't wear the same style every day.

• **Wear the right shoes.** If you're participating in athletic activities, wear the appropriate type of shoe for the sport.

• **Check shoes for wear and tear.** Replace or repair shoes when heels or insoles are worn.

• **Heed your heels.** If one heel is worn down more than the other, or shows greater wear on one side, it's a sign of an uneven gait. Check all your shoes to see whether it's that particular pair that's the problem. If not, a visit to a podiatrist can help.

• **Stay centered.** Wear backpacks and fanny packs centered on your back, not slung over one shoul-

SMART DEFINITION

Orthotics

Custom-made shoe inserts designed to correct foot abnormalities and improve gait and comfort, most often prescribed by a certified medical practitioner such as a podiatrist. Orthotics are also available without prescription by mail or on a variety of Web sites, from companies that custom-make inserts from at-home foot-impression kits. Follow-up by a podiatrist is highly recommended.

SMART MOVE

"When people test a new gadget, they usually feel better," said Richard Deyo, M.D., professor of medicine at the University of Washington, in an interview with *Time* magazine, noting that the effect often wears off before long, and the devices won't prevent another episode. "The one thing we know generally helps is exercise," said Dr. Deyo. "However, this requires exertion, not passive gadgets."

der or hanging down your side. Don't load up more than twenty pounds. If you must carry your wallet in a pants pocket, use a front pocket instead of the back to keep from sitting lopsided and twisting your spine.

Exercise Videos

As we've said throughout this book, when it comes to methods of back pain relief and prevention, exercise is top on the list. If you're thinking of using a video to help you, remember to take things slow. Those programs that emphasize stretching and flexibility, low-impact aerobics, and gentle strengthening are best. Stay away from jarring movements, and all those "iron man" routines.

"Anyone that talks biceps and triceps, and anaerobic and aerobic can look like an expert," says John Abdo, a certified fitness trainer with the International Sports Sciences Association and author of *Body Engineering*. Having a vocabulary is not the same as having knowledge, and jargon-laden instruction can interfere with the ability to teach.

Look for videos led by certified fitness professionals who include timeouts for heart-rate checking and rest, and stress a balanced program of fitness. Select a level of training that suits you. And Abdo warns viewers of all exercise videos, television programs, and even exercise classes to proceed with caution:

"If someone's doing something fast and explosive, do it slow and controlled so your body can become accustomed to the movement first. Never compete with the other guy or gal who's jumping or bounding around and who's been doing this for years."

With videos, remember the pause button, and use it. Or follow along at a slower pace. And remember: exercising without proper warmup, cooldown, and stretching; overdoing it; using improper form; or not wearing the proper footwear can get you hurt.

Good Nights

Sleeping on your side or back—or at least starting out that way—can help prevent backache, but what you're sleeping on has a lot to do with back health as well. A worn or inappropriate mattress or the wrong pillows can have a big effect.

Mattresses

Everyone knows that the firmer the mattress, the better, right? Wrong. Although firm is generally the better choice, a mattress can be either too soft *or* too hard.

"Extra-firm beds probably cause more problems than they solve," says Michael Lavin of European Sleep Works in Berkeley, California, praised by one ergonomist as the man who "knows more about mattresses than anybody in the country." Lying on a too-firm surface in most positions will force the body to hold its muscles rigid to support the spine.

"The absence of sag is more important than firmness," says Lavin. "A bed that sags in the middle creates different biomechanics that can be harmful to your back." Indeed, one of the advantages of firmer mattresses is not the firmness itself, but that

SMART SOURCES

Portable enough to use at the office or in the car, the BackCycler is like a lumbar support with a mind of its own. Automatically inflating and deflating on a two-minute cycle to exercise the lower spine even while you are sitting for hours, it can prevent or relieve stiffness and fatigue. Marketed in several models, from the basic, which provides about two inches of inflation, to a prescription-only version with up to six inches of lift, the Back-Cycler is available through its manufacturer and at most back-care stores for $99 to $349.

Ergonomics Inc.
800-959-3746

F.Y.I.

There are hourglass-shaped coils, individually pocketed springs, triple-offset sense-and-respond coils, and many more. But, according to *Consumer Reports,* there "simply aren't" any bad springs on sleep sets starting at around $450 for a twin-size set, $600 for a full-size, $800 for a queen-size, and $1,000 for a king-size. Based on their tests, neither coil design nor coil count affected quality or durability in any but the cheapest mattresses.

they will maintain their structure for a longer period of time.

Of course, too firm for one person might be just right for another. Individual differences in our body weight and form matter. A curvaceous, one-hundred-twenty-pound woman may barely "dent" one mattress, while a more linear, two-hundred-pound man might sink in.

Although the traditional innerspring mattress—coiled steel springs sandwiched between layers of padding—remains the most popular, many people opt for foam mattresses, water beds, and other types. Foam mattresses should be made of high-density foam, preferably natural latex, which not only can provide good support but is three to four times as durable as polyurethane foams.

Water beds, which can often be adjusted from what we call "stormy seas" to "waveless," appeal to a great number of back pain sufferers, who also enjoy the soothing warmth offered by heated models.

As for those adjustable beds we see advertised on late-night TV, the claims just don't measure up with reality. Elevating yourself into certain positions can increase pressure on the lumbar-sacral spine. While it might provide you some minutes of relief while you're changing position, over the long term it won't do much good.

Smart Advice on Mattresses

• Whatever you choose, remember that the most important thing is that the mattress is comfortable for you (check the warranty to be sure you'll have time to decide). And while a good bed is worth the investment, there's nothing wrong with shopping around for the right price.

"When you walk in and look for a mattress as the solution to your back pain, that sets up its own dynamic for overpricing," says Lavin. "It's a treacherous world, set up for charlatanism. Making extravagant claims and charging for it seems to be the modus operandi."

Furthermore, if small differences in the condition of the mattress make an extremely big difference to your back, it's probably not the mattress that's causing the pain.

• **Feel the firmness.** Don't rely on the label. The best mattress will support your body at all points. Orthopedic experts generally recommend the firmest mattress that you find comfortable. The wire in mattress springs comes in a range of thicknesses; the lower the gauge, the thicker and stiffer the wire, and the firmer the suspension.

• **Pass on the superplush padding.** In *Consumer Reports* tests, mattresses with thick, cushy padding tended to sag more, increasing the likelihood that you'll end up nestled in a slight indentation.

• **Buy the mattress and box spring at the same time.** They perform as a unit.

• **Put your feet up.** Some mattresses are more firm in some areas than in others. The middle might be firmer than the head or foot, or the edges might feature "extra support," for instance, to allow better "sitability." Different spring configurations may feel slightly different when you're sitting, but probably won't make much difference when you're lying down. See how it feels when you're in sleep position.

• **Don't be confused by jargon.** Mattresses are categorized into "quality levels" (such as premium,

SMART MOVE

"The addition of a one-inch thick piece of medium-density foam that costs about thirty dollars at a foam store might make more people feel better about their bed than anything I can think of," says Michael Lavin, of European Sleep Works. It also makes an easily transportable "travel pad." "You can roll it up and it doesn't take up too much room in the car."

superpremium, ultrapremium, or luxury), as well as firmness levels (pillow soft, plush, cushion firm, and superfirm), all of which vary by brand. One company's firm may be firmer than another's extra firm. You be the judge.

• **Separate but equal.** If you and your partner have significantly different mattress needs, consider a custom dual-sided mattress or the less-expensive option of two twin-size mattresses pushed together (accessories are available to fill the "crack").

• **Handle with proper care.** Watch for sags, and, to prolong its lifetime, turn your mattress over, and flip top to bottom at least four times a year.

Pillows, Headrests, Wedges

Nice, big, soft, fluffy pillows sure do sound great, but in reality they can be far from wonderful for your spine. At least if they're under your head: while two pillows are a definite no-no to lay your head upon, they can be a great help to your back if you place them elsewhere (see chapter 4).

A plethora of ergonomically designed pillows in a variety of shapes and materials is on the market today to support the curve of the neck and keep the spine properly aligned. Tailored for use during in-flight naps, while reading, or for sleeping in bed, the pillows keep you in a neutral position, anatomically, with your head straight, not bent. And if you just want to stick with your favorite standard pillow, a cervical roll inserted between it and the pillowcase can help reduce strain.

For the rest of the body, triangular foam wedges, some extending from thighs to feet, specifically designed to raise the knees and flatten the lumbar curve against the bed, can stay in place through the night when pillows won't. Another option: "night rolls" that tie around the waist.

Chairs

They're not just a few legs, a cushion, and a seat back anymore. Increasing numbers of furniture manufacturers are acknowledging the importance of ergonomics in the design of both office and home seating.

Herman Miller, a leader in the field of office furniture with more than a dozen chair designs in museums around the world, spends millions of dollars annually on ergonomic seating research. The company's Ergon chair, introduced in 1976, is considered the world's first ergonomic office chair, and it sold millions. In 1984, the Equa chair was named by *Time* magazine as one of the three "Best of the Decade" products of the eighties, along with the Apple Macintosh and the Mazda Miata. Launched in 1994, the futuristic-looking Aeron chair, in the permanent collection of New York's Museum of Modern Art, has been popularized by film and TV as the standard to which other chairs can only aspire.

"The vast bulk of sales are to large organizations, and they're buying them by the thousands," says Herman Miller's Mark Schurman. "Corporate America and international corporations are clearly buying these products because they see it as an issue of health, safety, productivity, employee morale, and retention. Shifts change but the chairs do not, so adjustable seating helps."

SMART SOURCES

Herman Miller, Inc.
616-654-3000
www.hermanmiller.com

Steelcase, Inc.
616-247-2710
www.steelcase.com

Haworth, Inc.
616-393-3000
www.haworth.com

Steelcase and Haworth are two other manufacturing leaders in the ergonomic office-furniture world.

On the other end of the scale can be found the less-conventional-looking Balans chairs, those strange-appearing backless seats with knee rests that are reputed to give the body a natural and more functional posture than traditional seating. The forward-slanting seat is designed to maintain proper alignment of the spinal column and reduce strain to the back. By allowing the sitter to lean forward with a straight back instead of having to hunch, the angle is also credited with preventing neck and shoulder problems. Some versions of kneeling chairs have a wheel base, while others use runners for more of a rocking motion.

On all manner of models, adjustable lumbar support, forward-tilt, movable cervical pillows, knee-tilt control, and anatomically contoured seats are just a few of the features offered today. Movable arm rests, rocking capability, and extra-tall backs are some other possibilities. Some offer "seat sliders" that, by moving forward and back, allow you to change the seat's depth for different tasks or different users.

Some back chairs are even portable, allowing you to transport your proper seating to the ballpark or beach. Home seating counts, too. One recliner boasts a combination of classic design with anatomical engineering. "This physician-recommended position," the catalog reads, "used by NASA astronauts during liftoff, promotes total relaxation by reducing physical stress. (Don't forget to attach your Reader's Window patented overhead book holder before blastoff.)

Whatever chair you choose should depend on where and how you'll be using it—as well as how long you'll be seated for when you use the chair—and what's comfortable for you. (See chapter 4 for more about back-healthy sitting positions).

Internet Caveat

Not only a major provider of back-pain-relief products, the Internet can provide a wealth of information on the subject. Just plug a key word into your search engine of choice, and you're off. Some Web sites allow you to download information for free that you'd have to pay for if you requested it by mail; others grant access to material otherwise available only to members.

Remember that anyone can put anything they want on the Internet, so stick with reputable, established sites. One of the first structured reviews of back pain resources on the Internet found only a minority offering unbiased, evidence-based information. "Most could be classified as advertisements, promoting a product or service related to back pain treatment," says Linda Li, P.T., who led the study, commissioned by the Institute for Work and Health in Toronto, Ontario.

A good general guide: sites ending in ".edu" are usually universities; ".gov" indicates government sites; and ".org" denotes nonprofit organizations. And watch for blatant commercialism wherever you are.

"The most important thing is to check out the credibility of the Web site sponsor," says Li, a physiotherapist who's noticed more and more patients bringing Internet printouts to therapy sessions. "It's similar to information from TV, or any form of the media—you have good sources of information

F.Y.I.

Of seventy-four back pain Web sites reviewed . . .

47 percent
Sponsored by for-profit companies

24.3 percent
Produced by nonprofit organizations

20.3 percent
Sponsored by health care providers

38.4 percent
Offered evidence-based information

9 sites
Classified as high quality

Source: "Surfing for Back Pain Sufferers: The Nature and Quality of Back Pain Information on the Internet," L. Li et al., Institute for Work and Health, Toronto, Canada.

and bad sources. You can't trust everything you see out there." Among Li's favorites:

*   www.amerchiro.org (American Chiropractic Association Online)

*   wellweb.com/index/qbackpai.htm (Wellness-Web)

*   www.vh.org/Patients/IHB/Ortho/BackPatient/Contents.html (Virtual Hospital)

Remember: Some Web sites were designed by people with more computer than back care expertise, and others by back care professionals who lack computer finesse. Take the source of the advice into account.

There are no miracle cures for back pain, and the answer to permanent healing cannot be found in any store. But that doesn't mean there isn't hope. With moderate exercise, good posture and movement, a healthy lifestyle including sound nutrition and rest, and a relaxed attitude, we have the surest means of preventing and overcoming ache. Priceless and safe, these methods are the smartest you'll find for back health.

THE BOTTOM LINE

The wide variety of products available to ease our aching backs can make life a lot easier—and more comfortable—for many. Carefully eliminate the "miracle cures" and unproven gadgets and gizmos, and you are still left with a broad range of options.

Index

Books in the
Smart Guide™ series

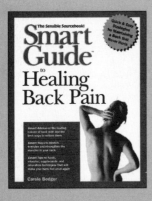
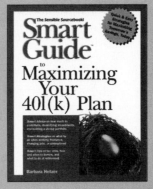
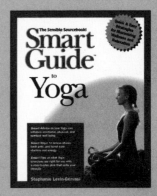

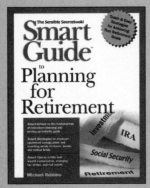
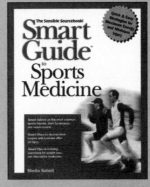
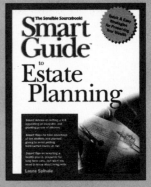